The Metamorphosis of the Mind

Transformative Insights for Winning the Battles of the Mind

Elisha O. Ogbonna

The Metamorphosis of the Mind: *Transformative Insights for Winning the Battles of the Mind*

by Elisha O. Ogbonna

Copyright © May 2024 by Elisha O. Ogbonna

All rights reserved. No part of this book may be reproduced, transmitted, or distributed in any form by any means, including, but not limited to, recording, photocopying, or taking screenshots of parts of the book, without prior written permission from the author or the publisher. Brief quotations for noncommercial purposes, such as book reviews, permitted by Fair Use of the Canada Copyright Law, are allowed without written permissions, as long as such quotations do not cause damage to the book's commercial value. For permissions, write to the publisher, whose address is stated below.

This book is written for educational and self-help purposes.

ISBN:
978-1-998457-01-4 (Hardcover)
978-1-998457-00-7 (Paperback)
978-1-7781320-9-4 (eBook)

Manufactured in Canada

Prinoelio Press
For Elisha Ogbonna
https://www.elishaogbonna.com

Dedication

Anthonia Onyenuwe,
whose inquiry in the year 2000 sparked the inception of my journey in exploring this subject.

Table of Contents

Dedication

Table of Contents

Introduction   9

CHAPTER 1

Psychological Perspectives on the Mind   13

CHAPTER 2

Philosophical Analysis of the Mind   25

CHAPTER 3

Theological Context of the Mind   37

CHAPTER 4

The Pith of the Human Conscious Mind   49

CHAPTER 5

The Essence of Unconscious Mind   55

CHAPTER 6

The District of Subconscious Mind   59

CHAPTER 7
The Five Powers of the Mind … 65

CHAPTER 8
The Five Laws of the Mind … 85

CHAPTER 9
The Stimuli of the Human Mind … 101

CHAPTER 10
The Shadows of Doubt and Insecurity … 109

CHAPTER 11
The Echoes of Guilt and Shame … 115

CHAPTER 12
The Spectrum of Anxiety and Paranoia … 121

CHAPTER 13
The Shadows of Depression … 129

CHAPTER 14
The Abyss of Suicidal Thoughts … 145

CHAPTER 15

Strategies for Winning the Internal Wars 159

CHAPTER 16
The Metamorphosis Stages and Processes 169

CHAPTER 17
Five Keys to Boosting Your Mind 203

CHAPTER 18
The Spiritual Dimensions of Mental Wellness 219

EPILOGUE 231

Introduction

Our minds operate much like the ebb and flow of day and night, often beyond our immediate control. They are like playgrounds where the forces of light and darkness converge, engaging in a persistent push for dominance and control. Like the varied activities found on a playground—seesaws, swings, and slides—our thoughts navigate through a multitude of experiences and learnings, shaped by our upbringing, life events, personal struggles, and personal beliefs. These interactions transform the landscape of our minds, changing them from arenas of play and innovativeness to battlegrounds of internal conflict and external stimuli.

In our world where the human mind grapples with many life challenges and the weight of failure, rejection, pain, disappointment, guilt, shame, insecurity, depression, suicidal thoughts, trauma, and other mental challenges, this guide is necessary for helping us understand defeating situations in our life, work, and relationships.

The phrase "metamorphosis of the mind" is metaphorical and often describes a profound and transformative change in one's thinking, beliefs, perceptions, or overall cognitive processes. This metaphor draws inspiration from the biological process of metamorphosis, where a creature undergoes a radical transformation in its form and structure. In the context of the mind, this transformation may involve shifts in consciousness, self-awareness, values, and perspectives. The metamorphosis of the mind represents a profound and transformative change in the way individuals think, perceive the world, and understand themselves. It's a dynamic process that involves self-reflection, learning, and a willingness to embrace new perspectives, ultimately leading to personal growth and a more nuanced understanding of the complexities of life.

The human mind, a complex region within the vast expanse of the human soul, has captivated thinkers, scholars, and seekers of understanding for centuries. In our quest to unravel the mysteries of this complex faculty, three major branches of study—psychology, philosophy, and theology—have emerged as beacons illuminating the intricate nature and functions of the human mind. However, amidst the wealth of descriptions and explanations provided by these disciplines, a critical examination reveals varying perspectives shaped by unique principles and conceptual frameworks.

"The Metamorphosis of the Mind" is a meticulously crafted guide designed to lead you through the intricate landscapes of the human mind. This transformative journey transcends conventional boundaries, delving deep into the multifaceted realms of psychology, philosophy, and theology. Its foundation is laid upon the pillars of psychological insights, philosophical reflections, and theological postulations, offering practical and transformative insights in your quest to conquer the internal battles that shape your existence.

For those who have felt the relentless grip of darkness, this book is a roadmap to not just navigate the shadows but to emerge victorious in the battles within. It extends its hand to individuals burdened by the weight of their minds, offering profound insights and practical strategies to transform pain into power, disappointment into resilience, and insecurity into unwavering self-assurance.

This isn't merely a collection of words; it's a lifeline for those who have weathered the storms within. As we navigate the triptych perspectives on the mind—psychological, philosophical, and theological—these pages unfold into a sanctuary of understanding. It's a space where the triad nature of the mind—conscious, unconscious, and subconscious—is explored, unraveling the mysteries that lie beneath the surface.

"The Metamorphosis of the Mind" extends a compassionate hand to those who have faced the shadows of depression and complex episodes of despair. Through the exploration of laws governing the mind, the potent arsenal within, and the revelation of strategies for emerging from the abyss of suicidal thoughts, this guide becomes a guardian for those seeking liberation.

The architects of thought, beliefs, and values are examined to uncover how they shape our mindscapes. Within this exploration, we learn the function of intuition and its potential to guide us out of the entanglements of our thoughts. With a focus on mental resilience, cognitive liberation, and perpetual metamorphosis, this book becomes a companion for those seeking a profound shift in their mental landscape.

To the reader carrying the burdens of the mind, this book is not just a source of knowledge; it is a lifeline, a guide, and a testament to the strength that resides within. As we journey through the chapters, we equip ourselves with the tools to face internal wars, stimulate the mind's symphony of awakening, and embrace perpetual transformation.

These pages will be a catalyst for metamorphosis, a source of inspiration, and a steadfast companion on the path to conquering the battles of the mind and emerging victorious in the pursuit of lasting well-being.

Chapter 1

Psychological Perspectives on the Mind

Psychology of the mind refers to the scientific study of the human mind and its functions. It encompasses a wide range of topics including perception, cognition, attention, memory, emotion, motivation, personality, and intelligence, among others. The field of psychology explores the nature of the mind and its relationship to the brain and body from various theoretical perspectives. There are several key concepts and theories within psychology that attempt to understand the intricacies of the mind-body relationship. Below are explanations of these concepts and theories:

Psychologists use various research methods such as experiments, surveys, and case studies, to investigate the functioning of the mind and brain. They study the brain through techniques such as brain imaging and brain stimulation, and they also use self-report measures and behavioral observations to gather information about the subjective experiences of individuals.

1. Cognitive Psychology: Cognitive psychology focuses on mental processes such as perception, memory, thinking, problem-solving, and language. It views the mind as an information-processing system, like a computer. In this perspective, the brain is the physical organ responsible for executing cognitive processes, and the mind is the product of these processes.

2. Biological Psychology (Biopsychology): Biological psychology examines the physiological basis of behavior and mental processes. It emphasizes the role of the nervous system, brain structures, neurotransmitters, and genetics in shaping the mind. According to this approach, mental states and processes are directly influenced by the physical properties and activities of the brain and body.

3. Behavioral Psychology: Behavioral psychology focuses on observable behaviors and the environmental factors that influence them. While it doesn't directly address the nature of the mind, it suggests that behaviors are learned responses to stimuli. The mind is often conceptualized as a black box, and the emphasis is on understanding and modifying observable behaviors.

4. Psychodynamic Psychology: Psychodynamic theories, particularly those developed by Sigmund Freud, propose that the mind consists of conscious and unconscious elements. The unconscious mind, shaped by early experiences and conflicts, influences behavior. The brain is seen as the physical organ, and the mind encompasses both conscious and unconscious mental processes. Psychodynamic theory, developed by Sigmund Freud, proposes that unconscious conflicts and experiences from childhood influence behavior and mental activity in adulthood.

5. Humanistic Psychology: Humanistic psychology emphasizes subjective experience, personal growth, and self-actualization. It views the mind as an active, purposeful entity seeking to fulfill its potential. The relationship between the mind and the brain is considered complex, with the mind influencing the brain's functioning and vice versa.

6. Cognitive Neuroscience: Cognitive neuroscience combines principles from cognitive psychology and neuroscience to investigate the neural basis of mental processes. It seeks to identify specific brain regions and neural mechanisms associated with cognitive functions such as perception, attention, and memory. Cognitive neuroscience combines neuropsychology and cognitive psychology to study the neural basis of mental processes and behavior. Cognitive development theory, most famously developed by Jean Piaget, explains how children's developmental processes such as perception, memory, and problem-solving throughout childhood.

7. Evolutionary Psychology: Evolutionary psychology posits that the mind has evolved to solve adaptive problems faced by human ancestors. It explores how psychological traits and processes might be shaped by natural selection. The brain is considered the physical organ that has evolved to support these adaptive mental processes. According to evolutionary psychology, the mind has evolved gradually through natural selection, leading to the emergence of specific mental processes and traits that aid in our survival and reproduction.

8. Social Psychology: Social psychology explores how individuals are influenced by social interactions and societal factors. It considers the role of social and cultural context in shaping the mind. The relationship between the mind and the body is often studied in the context of social influences on mental health and well-being.

Social learning theory proposes that people learn new behaviors by observing and imitating others. It also considers the role of reinforcement and punishment in shaping behavior.

9. Neuropsychology: Neuropsychology investigates how brain damage or dysfunction can affect cognitive functions and behavior. It helps establish correlations between specific brain areas and mental processes, shedding light on the relationship between the mind and the brain's structural and functional aspects. Neuropsychology views the mind as a product of the brain's anatomy and function. It explores the relationship between specific brain regions and cognitive functions, such as perception, memory, and language.

10. Ecological Psychology: Ecological psychology emphasizes the relationship between an individual and their environment. It considers how perception and action are coordinated in a particular context. The mind is viewed as an adaptive system that is closely connected to the environment in which it operates.

The Theory of Structuralism
Wilhelm Maximilian Wundt (1832—1920) was a physician, physiologist, philosopher, and professor. He exerted enormous influence on the development of psychology as a discipline and was able to distinguish psychology as a science from philosophy and biology He was the first person ever to call himself a psychologist. He was then accredited as the father of scientific psychology. He is known today as one of the founders of modern psychology.

In 1879, Wilhelm Wundt began the first psychological laboratory in Leipzig, Germany. At the University of Leipzig, Germany,

Wundt founded a school of thought in psychology called structuralism. Structuralism is a theory of consciousness developed by Wilhelm Wundt and his student Edward Bradford Titchener. Structuralism sought to analyze the adult mind (defined as the total experience from birth to the present) in terms of the simplest definable components and then to find how these components fit together in complex forms.[1]

The tenets of Wundt's school of thought were based on the agreement that psychology should begin its study of the mind in terms of elements that compose the structure of the mind. The structural school of thought believes that the structure of consciousness is composed of three major elements: sensations, images, and feelings which are elements of perceptions, elements of ideas, and elements of emotions respectively. Structuralism was based on introspection (i.e. technique of precise and rigorous self-examination). Titchener used introspection as a tool to determine the different components of human consciousness. He held that an experience should be classified as a fact, as it exists without any methodical examination of the significance or importance of that experience. Reliance on introspection got Titchener into trouble. This is because he believed that the "anatomy of the mind" had little to do with how or why the mind functions. Despite E.B. Titchener's (1867–1927) efforts, introspection failed to demonstrate objectivity, leading to a significant decline in the influence of the structural school of psychology after Titchener's death. Many psychologists opted for more objective methods instead.

---

[1] https://www.britannica.com/science/structuralism-psychology

The Theory of Functionalism
Functionalism is a theory of the mind that focuses on the functions and processes of mental states rather than their underlying physical structures. Unlike some other theories that emphasize the specific material or neurological aspects of the mind, functionalism is more concerned with how mental processes contribute to the overall functioning and adaptation of an organism.

William James (1842 – 1910) and John Dewey (1859 – 1952) supported functionalism. William James was an American philosopher and psychologist, and the first educator to offer a psychology course in the United States. James is considered to be a leading thinker of the late nineteenth century, one of the most influential philosophers of the United States, and the "Father of American psychology". He is the founder of the psychological movement of functionalism.

John Dewey, an American philosopher, psychologist, and educational reformer, has had a profound influence on education and social reform. He is regarded as one of the most prominent American scholars of the first half of the twentieth century. He was a founder of the philosophical movement known as pragmatism and a pioneer of functionalism.

Functionalism is a description of the theory of the mind that affirms that mental states are constituted solely by their functional role. This functional role includes their causal relations with other mental states, sensory inputs, and behavioral outputs. James and Dewey asserted that psychology should concern itself with the function of consciousness instead of the structure of consciousness. As a result, structuralism was then replaced by functionalism, which emphasized what the mind does rather than what it is composed of.

Here's an explanation of the nature of the mind and its relationship to the brain and body according to the theory of functionalism:

1. Emphasis on Function: Functionalism places a primary emphasis on the functions of mental processes rather than on the physical structures that may give rise to them. It's concerned with what the mind does, how it operates, and how mental processes contribute to an organism's ability to adapt and survive in its environment.

2. Adaptive Purpose: According to functionalism, mental states have an adaptive purpose in helping an organism interact with its environment. Mental processes are seen as mechanisms that enable an organism to perceive, learn, problem-solve, and respond to challenges in ways that enhance its chances of survival and reproduction.

3. Multiple Realizability: One key idea in functionalism is the concept of multiple realizability. This means that a particular mental function or state can be realized by various physical structures. In other words, different organisms or even artificial systems might have different neurological or physical configurations but still exhibit the same functional mental processes.

4. Focus on Behavior: Functionalism often looks at observable behavior as a key indicator of mental processes. The emphasis is on how mental states contribute to an organism's behavior and how different mental processes are related to each other in achieving a goal or responding to a stimulus.

5. Role of Inputs and Outputs: Functionalism considers the inputs (stimuli from the environment) and outputs (behavioral responses) associated with mental processes. The focus is on how the mind processes information from the environment and produces appropriate responses to achieve specific goals.

6. Mental States as Computations: Functionalism sometimes adopts a computational view of the mind, treating mental processes as information processing functions. In this sense, the mind is likened to a computer that takes inputs, processes information and produces outputs in a way that is functionally relevant to the organism's goals.

7. Holism: Functionalism tends to take a holistic approach to the mind, viewing mental processes as interrelated components that work together to support overall cognitive function. It is interested in understanding the mind as a system rather than focusing on isolated mental components.

8. Dynamic and Context-Dependent: The functionalist view acknowledges that mental processes can be dynamic and context-dependent. Mental states are seen as flexible responses to the ever-changing environment, and their functions may vary depending on the context in which they occur.

9. Technology and Artificial Intelligence: Functionalism has influenced the philosophy of mind in the context of artificial intelligence. It suggests that creating intelligent systems doesn't necessarily require replicating the exact structure of human brains but rather implementing functional processes that achieve similar goals.

In summary, functionalism sees the mind as a collection of processes that serve specific functions related to an organism's adaptation and survival. It is less concerned with the specific physical substrate of mental processes and more focused on how these processes contribute to an organism's behavior and interaction with its environment. The theory is particularly interested in the dynamic, purposeful nature of mental states and how they contribute to the overall functioning of an organism.

The theory Behaviourism
John Broadus Watson (1878 – 1958) was an American psychologist who popularized the scientific theory of behaviorism, establishing it as a psychological school. Watson advanced this change in the psychological discipline through his 1913 address at Columbia University, titled Psychology as the Behaviorist Views It. Watson objected to the tenets of functionalism because functionalism still accepted introspection (i.e. technique of precise and rigorous self-examination). This gave birth to the movement of behaviorism. Although Watson initially accepted instincts as important in explaining human behavior, he finally derived their influence. Behavior seen as instinctive, he argued, results from learning. He concluded that inheritance contributed little to behavior.

While behaviorism may seem intriguing, it has its flaws. For example, behaviorism asserts that once the stimulus is controlled, predicting the response becomes straightforward. However, this assertion may apply to lower animals but not to man. This is because humans are rational beings who may refuse to respond to any stimulus no matter what they need to do. Therefore, the stimulus-response theory of behavior propounded by J.B. Watson falls short in explaining all behaviors experienced in all humans. Also, the behaviors of human beings are not mechanical because human beings process information before acting. Consequently, studying the behaviors of individuals alone without paying attention to what goes on in the individual's mind is deficient.

The above three psychological approaches to the human mind's description appear not to completely explain the entirety of the mind in a concise statement or theory. As a result, let us delve into the other two branches of studies beginning with the philosophical position in the human mind's description.

One of the key goals of the psychology of the mind is to understand how the mind processes and interprets information from the world around us, as well as how it generates our thoughts, feelings, and behaviors. This includes understanding how we perceive and understand our environment, how we make decisions and form beliefs, and how our emotions influence our behavior.

Another important aspect of the psychology of the mind is the study of mental disorders and the development of effective treatments for these conditions. This involves understanding the underlying causes of mental disorders, as well as the neural, cognitive, and behavioral processes that are involved.

Overall, the psychology of the mind intends to provide a deep understanding of the workings of the human mind and its role in shaping our experiences and behavior. This knowledge can be applied to a wide range of fields, including education, healthcare, and social policy, to promote well-being and improve the quality of life for individuals and communities.

THE METAMORPHOSIS OF THE MIND

Chapter 2

Philosophical Analysis of the Mind

The philosophy of the mind is a branch of philosophy that deals with the nature of the mind, consciousness, and the relationship between the mind and the body. It aims to answer questions such as, "What is the mind?" "What is consciousness?" and "How is the mind related to the body?"

Philosophers of the mind have proposed a variety of theories to answer these questions, ranging from materialism, which holds that the mind is simply a product of the brain and body, to dualism, which argues that the mind and body are distinct entities. Other prominent theories include functionalism, which views the mind as a set of mental states and processes, and idealism, which holds that the mind is the source of all reality.

The Theory of Materialism:
Materialism is a philosophical stance that asserts that everything that exists is composed of material or physical substance and that mental phenomena, such as thoughts, consciousness, and the mind, are ultimately the result of physical processes. In the context of the mind and its relationship to the brain and body, materialism posits that mental states and processes are entirely dependent on and can

be explained by the physical properties and activities of the brain and the body.

1. Fundamental Assumption: Materialism starts with the fundamental assumption that everything in the universe, including the mind, can be reduced to and explained by the physical components that make it up. In the case of the mind, this means that mental phenomena are considered to be a product of the physical structure and processes of the brain.

2. Identity Theory: One specific form of materialism related to the mind-body problem is identity theory. Identity theory proposes that mental states are identical to specific brain states. In other words, mental events and processes are just different ways of describing the same underlying physical reality in the brain.

3. Reductionism: Materialism often involves a reductionist approach, aiming to reduce complex mental phenomena to simpler, more fundamental physical processes. For instance, emotions, thoughts, and consciousness are seen as ultimately being reducible to the activity of neurons, neurotransmitters, and other physical components of the brain.

4. Causation: Materialism asserts that mental events and states are caused by and are causally linked to physical events and states. Changes in the physical state of the brain are believed to directly cause changes in mental states, and vice versa. This causal relationship is central to understanding how materialists view the interaction between the mind and the brain.

5. *No Dualism:* In contrast to dualism, which posits a mind-body duality, materialism insists that the mind is a product of the physical processes of the body and, more specifically, the brain.

6. *Neuroscientific Evidence:* Materialists often rely on evidence from neuroscience to support their claims. Advances in neuroscience have allowed researchers to identify specific regions of the brain associated with various mental functions and observe how changes in brain activity correspond to changes in mental states. This empirical approach reinforces the materialist perspective.

7. *Emergence:* Some materialists acknowledge the concept of emergence, where complex mental phenomena emerge from the interactions of simpler physical components in the brain. While the mind is considered an emergent property of the brain, it is ultimately seen as being fully explainable by the physical properties of its constituent parts.

In summary, materialism asserts that the mind and its various aspects are entirely explicable through the physical components and processes of the brain and body. Mental states are nothing more than the result of complex physical interactions, and the mind is ultimately reducible to and dependent upon the material substance of the brain. This perspective contrasts with dualism, which posits a fundamental distinction between the mental and the physical.

The theory of Dualism
Dualism is a philosophical stance that posits a fundamental distinction between the mind and the body. According to dualism, the mind and the body are two ontologically distinct entities, each

with its unique characteristics and properties. This perspective stands in contrast to monism, which asserts that there is only one fundamental substance or reality. Dualism can take various forms, but the most common distinction is between the mental (mind) and the physical (body). Here's an explanation of the nature of the mind and its relationship to the brain and body according to the theory of dualism:

1. Mind-Body Distinction: Dualism begins with the fundamental idea that the mind and the body are separate and distinct entities. The mind is often associated with consciousness, thoughts, feelings, and subjective experiences, while the body is viewed as the physical, material aspect that includes the brain, organs, and other bodily tissues.

2. Interactionism: Dualism acknowledges that there is an interaction between the mind and the body, although the nature of this interaction is debated among dualists. Interactionism proposes a two-way causal relationship between the mental and the physical: the mind can influence the body, and vice versa. However, how this interaction occurs without violating the laws of physics remains a challenging question.

3. Substance Dualism: Substance dualism is a specific form of dualism that asserts the existence of two fundamentally different substances: mental substance (mind or soul) and physical substance (body). According to this view, the mind and the body are separate substances that exist independently. René Descartes, a prominent philosopher, is often associated with substance dualism.

4. Epistemic Dualism: Another form of dualism is epistemic dualism, which doesn't necessarily posit two distinct substances but emphasizes a fundamental epistemological distinction. It suggests that the mind and the body are known in different ways or have different kinds of properties that cannot be fully understood through the same methods.

5. Property Dualism: Property dualism asserts that mental properties and physical properties are irreducible to each other but do not necessarily imply the existence of distinct substances. Mental properties, such as consciousness, cannot be fully explained or reduced to physical properties, such as neural activity.

6. Non-Reductionism: Dualism is often associated with non-reductionism, meaning that mental phenomena are not reducible to, or explainable solely by, physical processes. This stands in contrast to materialism, which aims to explain mental phenomena exclusively in terms of physical processes.

Critiques of Materialism: Dualism often arises as a response to perceived shortcomings of materialist theories in explaining consciousness, subjective experience, and the nature of the self. Dualists argue that these aspects of the mind cannot be adequately accounted for within a purely materialistic framework.

Afterlife and Immortality: Some dualistic views incorporate the idea of an immortal soul or consciousness that persists beyond the death of the physical body. The separation of the mind from the body in dualism can lead to philosophical discussions about the nature of life, death, and the possibility of an afterlife.

In summary, according to dualism, the mind and the body are distinct entities with different properties, and their relationship involves some form of interaction. The specific form of dualism (substance, property, epistemic) may vary, but all dualistic theories reject the idea that mental phenomena can be fully explained in terms of physical processes alone. The mind, in the dualistic view, retains a unique and irreducible status.

The Theory of Pluralism:
Pluralism is a philosophical viewpoint that holds that many underlying substances make up human brains and bodies. Pluralism proposes that several fundamental elements are influencing human existence, in contrast to monism, which maintains that there is only one fundamental material. Pluralism accommodates the notion that different people may have unique mixtures of fundamental substances, leading to variations in mental and physical characteristics. Recognizing these differences makes understanding the uniqueness of individuals easier.

Philosophical disputes regarding memory sometimes center on the nature of memory itself—whether it is essentially a mental construct formed by cognitive processes or the result of complex physiological interactions. Since pluralism recognizes the merits of both points of view, it offers a framework for having these discussions. Hybrid viewpoints that combine aspects of other philosophical stances, like monism or dualism, are frequently welcomed into pluralism. This adaptability makes it possible to comprehend the complexity of the human experience in a more inclusive and nuanced way. Here's a look at some of the fundamental principles of pluralism:

Diverse Substances: Pluralism contends that the minds and bodies of humans are composed of a variety of basic substances rather than a single, unified substance. These diverse elements contribute to the complexity and richness of human experience. Pluralism often encourages a holistic understanding of human beings, considering the diverse substances as integral components of a unified whole. This holistic approach recognizes the interconnectedness of the different elements within the human experience.

Mind-Body Distinction: Pluralism often recognizes a clear distinction between the mind and the body, with each having its unique set of basic substances. This separation allows for a nuanced understanding of the mental and physical aspects of human existence. Pluralism suggests that the various substances interacting within the mind and body influence each other. The dynamic interplay among these substances contributes to the complexity of human behavior, emotions, and thought processes. In pluralistic perspectives, the relations between mental and physical phenomena are intricate and involve the intermingling of diverse substances. This view allows for a more nuanced exploration of the mind-body relationship.

Pluralism emphasizes the dynamic interaction between the mind and body in the process of memory. The cognitive act of remembering is intricately connected to the physiological processes occurring in the brain, illustrating the collaboration between mental and physical substances.

Multifaceted Consciousness: According to pluralism, consciousness arises from a combination of different substances, each contributing to various facets of cognitive and experiential processes. This multifaceted approach offers a comprehensive view of the nature of consciousness. Different individuals may exhibit variations in their memory abilities, reflecting unique combinations of cognitive and biological factors. Some individuals might excel in recalling factual information, highlighting the diversity in the cognitive substances contributing to memory.

The Cognitive and Biological Elements of Memory: In the context of memory, pluralism can be exemplified by considering the diverse substances that contribute to the complex phenomenon of remembering. Memory involves both cognitive and biological elements, showcasing the interconnectedness and multifaceted nature of human experience. Pluralism acknowledges that memory is not solely a result of one cognitive substance but involves various mental processes. For instance, declarative memory, which involves the recall of facts and events, may be supported by different cognitive mechanisms than procedural memory, which pertains to skills and habits.

From a pluralistic perspective, the biological basis of memory includes a combination of substances within the brain. Synaptic connections, neurotransmitters, and specific brain regions all contribute to the formation, consolidation, and retrieval of memories. Each of these elements represents a distinct biological substance.

Some forms of pluralism extend beyond the realm of mind and body to encompass a broader philosophical perspective. This may involve recognizing diverse fundamental substances in the broader context of metaphysics or ontology.

In summary, pluralism asserts that there is a plurality of basic substances shaping the minds and bodies of humans. This perspective embraces diversity and complexity, providing a framework for understanding the intricate interplay of various elements within the human experience.

The theory of Idealism
Idealism is a philosophical perspective that posits the primacy of ideas, consciousness, or mind as fundamental in the constitution of reality. In the context of the mind, idealism asserts that the mind is not a product of the physical brain but is the foundational reality, and the physical world, including the body and the brain, is a manifestation or appearance of the mind. Here's an explanation of the nature of the mind and its relationship to the brain and body according to the theory of idealism:

1. Primacy of Mind: Idealism holds that the mind is primary, and it asserts that reality is fundamentally mental or consciousness-based. In contrast to materialism, which claims that the mind arises from physical processes, idealism asserts that the physical world, including the brain and body, is a product or projection of the mind.

2. Epistemological Idealism: Some forms of idealism focus on epistemology, emphasizing that the nature of reality is dependent on perception and consciousness. According to this view, reality exists as it is known or perceived, and the mind plays a central role in shaping and defining what is real.

3. *Non-Physical Nature of Mind:* Idealism rejects the notion that the mind is a physical entity, such as the brain. Instead, the mind is considered to be non-physical, existing in a realm beyond the

material world. The physical world, including the body and brain, is seen as a manifestation of the mind's activity.

4. Berkeleyan Idealism: A notable form of idealism is associated with the philosopher George Berkeley. Berkeleyan idealism argues that the material world exists only insofar as it is perceived by a conscious mind. The famous phrase "esse est percipi" (to be is to be perceived) encapsulates the idea that things exist because they are perceived.

5. Subjective Reality: Idealism often leads to a subjective understanding of reality because reality is perceived as dependent on the mind or consciousness. This means that different minds may experience different realities, as the external world's reality is considered contingent on the perceiving subject.

6. Immaterial Consciousness: Idealism suggests that consciousness or the mind is not a product of material processes. Instead, consciousness is considered to be immaterial, existing independently of the physical world. This immaterial consciousness is primary and gives rise to the apparent material reality.

7. Reality as Mental Constructs: Idealism views the external world, including the body and brain, as mental constructs or representations. The physical world is seen as a projection of the mind's activity rather than an independent, objective reality.

8. Unity of Mind and Reality: In idealism, there is a unity between the mind and reality. The distinction between the perceiver and the perceived are often blurred, and reality is understood as an integral part of the mind's activity.

9. Metaphysical Idealism: Some forms of idealism take a metaphysical stance, positing that the ultimate reality is a transcendent, universal mind or consciousness. In this view, individual minds are interconnected aspects of a greater, unified consciousness.

10 Challenges to Materialism: Idealism often emerges as a response to perceived challenges or limitations in materialistic explanations of consciousness and the mind. It challenges the notion that the mind can be entirely reduced to physical processes.

In summary, idealism posits that the mind is the fundamental reality, and the physical world, including the brain and body, is derived from or dependent on the mind. It offers a different perspective on the relationship between consciousness and the external world, emphasizing the centrality of mental processes in shaping our understanding of reality.

In contrast to psychology, the philosophy of the mind is more focused on the abstract and theoretical aspects of the mind and its relationship to the body and the world. It is concerned with questions of metaphysics, epistemology, and ethics, and it uses logic, argument, and reason to support its claims.

While the philosophy of the mind is concerned with broader questions about the nature of the mind and consciousness, the psychology of the mind is focused on empirical research and scientific investigation into the workings of the mind. It uses a range of research methods, including experiments, surveys, and brain imaging, to study the underlying processes and mechanisms of the mind, as well as its relationship to behavior and the environment.

The philosophy of the mind is concerned with the abstract and theoretical aspects of the mind and consciousness, while the psychology of the mind is focused on the empirical study of the mind and its functions. Both fields complement each other and play a crucial role in our understanding of the mind and its relationship to the world.

It is important to note that while these theories have different focuses and approaches, they are not necessarily mutually exclusive. In many cases, they can complement each other, providing a more comprehensive understanding of the mind and its functions. For example, a combination of neuropsychology and cognitive development theory can help us understand how brain development and experience interact to shape mental processes.

Many of these theories have practical applications in various fields. For example, social learning theory has been used to develop effective educational programs, while cognitive neuroscience has helped inform the development of new technologies and treatments for neurological disorders.

In conclusion, the study of the mind and its relationship to the brain is a complex and interdisciplinary field that draws from many areas of study, including psychology, biology, neuroscience, and philosophy. By considering multiple perspectives and theories, we can gain a deeper understanding of the mind and its functions, which can have important implications for our health and well-being.

Chapter 3

Theological Context of the Mind

Theology is the intellectual pursuit and systematic study of the nature of God and religious truths. It involves rational inquiry into questions related to religion and seeks to understand the attributes of God and His relationship to the universe. Theological inquiry is not limited to any specific religion but encompasses a broad spectrum of belief systems. In Christian theology, the Bible serves as the foundational text, offering insights into God's nature, His attributes, and the principles of Christianity.

Within the realm of theology, there is a specific branch called theological anthropology, which focuses on the study of humans about God. This field is distinct from social science anthropology, which looks into comparing the physical and social aspects of humanity across various cultures and times.

In the theological domain, the mind is considered not merely as a product of cognitive processes but as a divine gift intertwined with the spiritual essence of human existence. Theology, grounded in religious and spiritual traditions, posits that the mind is a conduit for divine connection and a vessel for transcendent experiences. Here, discussions delve into matters of morality, ethics, and the soul's journey toward enlightenment. As we delve into the theological perspectives on the mind, we will explore the profound intersections between faith, reason, and the transformative power of spiritual awakening.

In the theological domain, the contemplation of the mind transcends its mere function as a cognitive apparatus. Instead, theologians view the mind as a sacred endowment, intricately woven into the fabric of spiritual existence. Rooted in ancient religious and spiritual traditions, theology posits that the mind serves as more than a mechanism for processing information; it is a conduit through which individuals can forge a divine connection and access transcendent experiences.

1. *Divine Gift and Spiritual Essence*: According to theological perspectives, the mind is regarded as a divine gift, bestowed upon individuals as an integral part of their spiritual essence. This viewpoint suggests that the mind is not a random byproduct of evolution but a deliberate bestowal, a medium through which humans can engage with the sacred dimensions of existence. In this light, the mind is seen as a channel for divine communication, a bridge between the earthly and the divine.

2. *Conduit for Divine Connection*: Theological discussions on the mind emphasize its role as a conduit for divine connection. The mind, in this context, becomes a sacred instrument through which individuals can commune with the divine, seek guidance, and deepen their understanding of spiritual truths. It is through contemplation, prayer, and meditation that the mind is believed to facilitate a profound connection with the transcendent.

3. *Vessel for Transcendent Experiences*: Theology posits that the mind acts as a vessel for transcendent experiences, wherein

individuals may encounter moments of profound spiritual insight and revelation. Through prayerful reflection, mindfulness, and the cultivation of spiritual disciplines, the mind becomes receptive to experiences that transcend the boundaries of the material world, offering glimpses into the ineffable realms of the divine.

4. *Exploration of Morality and Ethics*: Within the theological discourse on the mind, discussions extend beyond cognitive processes to encompass matters of morality and ethics. The mind, regarded as a divine gift, is seen as a moral compass that guides individuals in their ethical deliberations and actions. The theological exploration of the mind engages with questions of right and wrong, virtue and sin, illuminating the ethical dimensions of human existence.

Thought is the attribute of the human mind's ability to process judgment, analyze, and synthesize knowledge and experience to determine the true value of an incident and guide you to develop an appropriate response. The biblical term for the right response is wit. Wit is the use of the right discretion to judge and define a thing. It is equivalent to wisdom. However, wisdom is the same thing as common sense or equivalent to the use of sense because where sense fails, wisdom continues. The scripture, wit, or soundness of mind connotes confidence, awareness, and good nature of the mind which enable it to analyze and critically look into an event and remove every element of compromise without being biased. In the above context, the Bible references it as rightness of mind.[2]

---

[2] see Mark 5:15; Luke 8:35.

5. *The Soul's Journey Towards Enlightenment*: Theological perspectives on the mind are intrinsically linked to the soul's journey towards enlightenment. The mind, as an ally to the soul, is seen as a vehicle for spiritual growth and transformation. The journey involves the purification of the mind through spiritual practices, leading to a heightened awareness of divine truths and a deeper connection with the transcendent.

6. *Intersections of Faith, Reason, and Spiritual Awakening*: As we delve into theological perspectives on the mind, we navigate the profound intersections of faith, reason, and the transformative power of spiritual awakening. Faith, grounded in belief systems, coexists with reason, encouraging a thoughtful exploration of spiritual truths. The amazing power of spiritual awakening shines through when people, by nurturing their minds, begin a journey of faith that goes beyond mere understanding, resulting in a deep transformation of the soul.

7. *The Memory, Affection, and the Will*: The mind is capable of recalling images or events and other episodes occurring at a particular time and place which creates in it an awareness that has a particular content. Several states of consciousness linked by memory are about the conscious states of the mind. The Bible expressed it in this form: 'I am forgotten as a dead man out of mind memory.[3] Remember, this brings it again to mind [memory].[4] Memory serves as the warehouse of the mind, constantly pressing upon the subconscious the events of significance or impact, which are then broadcasted into the human soul through the frequency

---

[3] Ps. 31:12.
[4] Isa. 46:8.

band of imagination, whether consciously or unconsciously. The import is dependent on the frequency of modulation and wavelength.

The scriptures recognize human will as a volitional attribute of the mind (soul). In depiction, it portrays it as where intellect and emotion are used together to produce a response to an event. The Bible word used is 'ready mind'.[5] Affection is the area of expression involving judgment and emotion for a particular response. Emotion gives our thought life and vitality. The fact remains, nobody would do a thing that they have not chosen to do and nobody. People do what they want to do when what happened to them is the reason for their actions. We may not deny the fact that sometimes the things that people do are either to impress or offend somebody. In terms of volition, when the human mind has rationalized an event and prepares itself for an action, it would engage the human will for action. The ready mind is willing. It has a combined effort that is determined to act.

In summary, the theological contemplation of the mind encompasses its divine origin, role as a conduit for connection and function as a vessel for transcendent experiences. The exploration extends into ethical considerations and the symbiotic relationship between the mind and the soul's journey towards enlightenment. The intersections of faith, reason, and spiritual awakening highlight the depth and richness of theological perspectives on the transformative nature of the human mind.

---

[5] 1 Peter 5:2

Metaphorical Theology Context of the Mind

Theology is the study of God and the existence of God. In theology, the greatest book is the Bible. The Bible is a book written by the inspiration of God. It has two parts, 66 books, and 40 writers over 1600 years. In the biblical context, the mind signifies the understanding, or good judgment, whereby we distinguish between good and evil, lawful and unlawful. The two adjectives to qualify this include blindness of the Mind[6] and defilement of the mind.[7]

In the Bible, *Blindness of the mind* is an expression that refers to the condition of the mind in which a person lacks perception, awareness, or judgment and as a result is ignorant of how they are, where they are and the things happening within and around them. This individual whose mind has been covered would not perceive things in their right form. *Defined mind* is a mind that is made unclean, either literally or figuratively. It results from distortion of truth which degenerates human conscience and impacts the mind with all sorts of unholy thinking and actions that may include diabolic, sinful, and selfish lust to the point of self-destruction.

In the above instances, the human mind is not seen as a physical thing, but an intangible aspect of human nature located in his inner being (soul) and used for moral reasoning and value analysis. The Holy Bible lays great emphasis on the spiritual thing, it revealed in the book of Titus that there is a liaison that exists between the mind and conscience which proves that the mind is the seat of judgment (reasoning) whereas the conscience does the function of giving the

---

[6] 2 Cor. 3:14, 4:4
[7] Titus 1:15

result of peace or trouble that is consequential to the action taken by one's choosing from such judgment (reasoning).

The mind in many biblical injunctions is referred to as the heart.[8] More often than not, the scriptures use the physical to describe the intangible. The scripture attributes of the physical heart are equivalent to the attributes of the mind to the human soul in terms of functions. For instance, the primary function of the human physical heart is to pump blood in the circulatory system, likewise, the mind (spiritual heart) pumps and distributes knowledge and judgment. The heart has four chambers—right auricle, left auricle, right ventricle, and left ventricle but the mind has the unconscious, conscious and subconscious (memory), and the imagination.

Like the philosophy of the mind, theologically, the scripture acknowledges the elements of inward human being cognitive, affective, and volition in terms of thought (and imagination), affection, and will. But unlike the philosophy of the mind, the scripture acknowledges them are attributes of the human soul.

The States of the Mind
The Bible has two major distinctive descriptions of the human mind. It described the mind as either the mind of the flesh or the mind of the spirit. This description places human action and behavior into two groups: spiritual mind (pure or holy thought) and carnal mind (corrupt, defiled, or unholy thought). The epistles of Apostle Paul to Roman chapter eight reveal that to be carnally minded is dead and to be spiritually minded is life. This shows a clear distinction represents the difference between light and

---

[8] Gen. 26:35, Deut. 18:6.

darkness, good and evil as well as life and death. Let's consider what constitutes carnal and spiritual-mindedness.

Carnal Mind/Mind of the Flesh
The carnal mind in the biblical context refers to a hostile, self-centered, and selfish state of the human mind. This is evident in the phrase "mind of the flesh" or "lust of the flesh". It does not apply to the physical desire of hunger and thirst including a call of nature that would in no way to advantage of others. In terms of spiritual and moral terms, we cannot make the flesh act right or bring it into obedience to the law of God by any means. Thus, flesh or fleshly desire is a biblical metaphor to describe sinful tendencies. Although the scripture recognizes human willpower, it does describe it as weak in doing tricks.

For instance, the use of willpower is compared to using the flesh to deal with fleshly desires which is stronger and more forceful. That means flesh in that context does not refer to the body (the physical structure of a human being). It is not the meat of the body but rather the urge, desire, lust, or vibration of thought that is generated by fleeting desires, undisciplined feelings, reasoning, and experiences. Feelings that do not agree with the divine instructions about life and moral living are the by-product of the carnal mind. Emotions that are remote-controlled by hormones, body chemistry, or lust and devoid of love are influenced by the "mind of the flesh". Feelings of sinful tendencies, that fan your ego promote your ungodly fantasy, and less likely to submit to willpower. The carnal mind produces carnal feelings that contradict truth and the way of truth. Feelings that tell you, you are up there whereas you are down here.

Other descriptive forms of carnal mind are doubtful/skeptical mind; feeble mind; Double mind; Proud mind; Hostile Mind; Wicked mind; Reprobate Mind; Corrupt Mind; Evil evil-affected mind; and Hardened Mind.[9] The three major driving forces of a carnal mind are the pride of life, the lust of the flesh, and the lust of the eyes.[10] This is confirmed by this scriptural quote: "For they that are after the flesh do mind the things of the flesh; but they that are after the Spirit the things of the Spirit. For to be carnally minded is death, but to be spiritually minded is life and peace."[11]

Spiritual Mind/Mind of the Spirit
Spirit mind worded as spiritually minded is a biblical metaphorical depiction of having a mind set on spiritual things---a mind filled with holy desires and purposes. The spirit in this context is capitalized and therefore does not refer to the human spirit which is referred to as "the candle of the Lord".[12] The mind of the Spirit refers to a mind that is in obedience to the leading of the Holy Spirit. The Holy Spirit empowers, enlightens, and brings to light the infinite knowledge and awareness of the human mind. Inspirations that are not accessible by the mind of the flesh can be obtained with the help of the Spirit.

The human spirit is often metaphorically referred to as the candle of the Lord, likened to the cognitive part of the human spirit (i.e. intuition) or soul (transformed mind). A candle when lighted produces light that drives away the darkness in the same manner

---

[9] Luke 12:29; 1 These. 5;14; James 1:8, 4:8; Col. 21:18; Act. 12:20; Pro. 21:27, Col. 1:21-22; Rom. 1:20; 1 Tim. 6:5; Act 14:2; Dan. 5:20.
[10] 1 John 2:16
[11] Romans 8:5.
[12] Pro. 20:27.

when the human spirit is enlightened and the mind renewed, they become strengthened to reason morally and observe and judge their actions amid sinful tendencies (carnally mindedness). Also, this individual would be able to see and recognize the gifts and graces which God has endowed him with, which are not given only for their sake, but for the good of others. This is supported by the scriptural expression, "Neither do men light a candle, and put it under a bushel, but on a candlestick, and it. giveth light unto all that are in the house."[13]

Other descriptive forms of carnal mind are sound mind; steady mind; willing mind; ready mind; one mind; humble mind; right Mind; and fervent mind.[14] The three major driving forces of a carnal mind are the spirit of love, the spirit of truth, and the spirit of life. The mind of the spirit is a transformed mind. It is a mind that has God's consciousness and desire to know His will and purpose and to follow them.

Transforming one's mind is the biblical recommendation for having and holding unto the mind of the Spirit. Unfortunately, the human mind cannot be born again just like the spirit. It does not experience an absolute new birth like the human spirit. A new birth is a spiritual event that produces a new spirit. Even with the new spirit, a person would have to fight the battle within their minds. This is why the scripture admonishes people to transform their lives by the daily

---

[13] Matt. 5:15.
[14] (2 Tim. 1:7); (Isa. 26:3); (1 Chron. 28:9); (Act 17:11, 1 Peter 5:2); (Rom. 12:16; Rom. 15:6; Phil. 4:2; 1 Peter 3:8); (Phil. 2;3; Act 20:19; Col. 3:12); (Mark 5:15); (2 Cor. 7:7).

renewal of their minds.[15] They do not have to fight fleshy desires with their carnal mind but by the spirit—the new spirit that is empowered and inspired by the Holy Spirit.

Why is mind renewal such a significant concept for believers? The scripture acknowledges that everyone, at some point or another, would be exposed to intrusive thoughts. These intrusive thoughts consist of involuntary thinking, unwanted images, words, phrases, or impulses that are extremely common in our environment. Our experiences and fleshly desires can subject us to spontaneous and intrusive thoughts, in this computer age where at a click of a button one can watch the news or read the horrible events happening around the globe. It is easy to be affected by the daily abuses and violence, inappropriate sexual displays, and people making jokes about God. Blasphemy can be extremely disturbing and even cause some to question the existence of God.

The scripture does not deny the existence of intrusive thoughts. This is why it has asked us to fight intrusive thoughts. It encourages us to submit our hearts and thoughts to God. The Holy Spirit can help us determine if there is anything harmful in our thoughts. He can help us deal with overpowering immoral thinking. Thoughts that are unbidden and spontaneous can be controlled by learning and studying a scriptural approach, reaffirming the truth of God's Word in our minds, and memorizing biblical quotes that build and energize our spirit. These alongside prayers can greatly diminish or even vanquish intrusive thoughts.

---

[15] Rom. 12:2

Intrusive thoughts, even those that are blasphemous, are not necessarily sinful. The human mind is a weak battleground for fleshly desires, and we can easily be influenced by the world and events around us. However, for anyone to intentionally expose themselves to immoral thoughts and other evils, they may be considered to have sinned. Another way of giving intrusive thoughts a foothold is by surrounding yourself with worldly things. The greater one is exposed to immoral and worldly things, the more those things will occupy our thoughts.

In summary, intrusive thoughts can emanate from chemical biological activities or the chemical imbalance of our physical body. An imbalance in a person's body's chemical activities may result in a symptom of depression, attention deficit disorder, and obsessive-compulsive disorder, among other things. This is why it is important to seek help and advice from professionals on these things as well as spiritual help in spiritual matters.

Chapter 4

The Pith of the Human Conscious Mind

The conscious mind refers to the aspect of our mental process that is aware of our thoughts, emotions, and surroundings. It is responsible for our ability to process information, make decisions, and direct our attention to the things we are focusing on. The conscious mind is only a small part of the workings of our minds.

When you read a book, for instance, your conscious mind is actively digesting the words, connecting the dots between the details, and developing a comprehension of the narrative. The unconscious processes that operate in the background, like your breathing and heartbeat, are not the same as this conscious processing.

The conscious mind is where we receive information, make decisions, and regulate our behavior. It can be viewed as the hub of our thoughts for making decisions. It is also in charge of our capacity for introspection and self-awareness regarding our feelings, ideas, and experiences.

It is crucial to remember that the conscious mind has a certain amount of processing power and can become overloaded if we attempt to multitask. This explains why, following a demanding workday or after studying for a test, we could feel mentally spent. It's critical to partake in relaxing and mindfulness-promoting activities, like meditation, or deep breathing exercises, to preserve healthy performance.

Another crucial aspect of the conscious mind is its capacity for training and development. Similar to how we can strengthen our physical muscles through exercise and training, we can enhance the functioning of our conscious mind through practices like mindfulness, visualization, and positive thinking. When we intentionally focus our attention on certain thoughts or activities, we can strengthen the connections between the neurons in our brain and improve the efficiency of our conscious mind.

It is also worth mentioning that the conscious mind and the unconscious mind are not separate entities but are rather interconnected and constantly influencing each other. For example, our unconscious beliefs and experiences can impact the way we perceive the world and the decisions we make, even if we are not consciously aware of these influences. On the other hand, our conscious thoughts and actions can shape and change our unconscious beliefs and behaviors over time.

The conscious mind can be explained in three analogies: the language tense analogy, the computer system analogy, and the refrigeration analogy. The conscious mind as the term applies represents the mental operation and experiences that we are attentive to and have full awareness of at the moment. It is the region of the mind where we think, judge, consider, or regard our thoughts and experiences.

In terms of language tenses, the conscious mind represents mental experiences in either the present tenses or present continuous tenses. Conscious minds are thoughts that exist in a tense expressing a mental experience that is currently going on or habitually performed, or a state of the mind that currently or generally exists. Present continuous tense indicates that an action or condition is happening now, frequently, and may continue, and so is the mental processing that defines the conscious mind.

The conscious mind is where our thoughts, memories, feelings, and desires are sorted, processed, and refined when we're aware of them and pay attention. It's part of our mind that systematically processes our thoughts and feelings by continuously organizing awareness and related information into coherent ideas that we can think and talk about logically. A part of this includes our imagination, which does the work of a magnifying lens and warehouse of creativity. Besides it is our memory comprising the subconscious and unconscious minds which although not always part of consciousness work alongside the conscious mind by bringing in the stored thoughts and experiences easily at any time into our awareness for our conscious mind usage.

The action of thinking about something in a logical, sensible way is accomplished with the conscious mind. However, the mind is not where all the actions of the mind take place. There is no question about using our conscious mind to rationalize events that we are aware of and reasonably talk about. When it comes to sensations, perceptions, memories, feelings, and fantasies inside of our currently unaware, other aspects of our minds take subliminal actions. Subliminal is a phenomenon of a stimulus or mental process that is below the threshold of sensation or consciousness. It is any of the unperceived or partially perceived mental processes that affect someone's mind without their being consciously aware of it.

When certain events and experiences that have been rationalized by the conscious mind become obsolete, less relevant, or unattended to the conscious mind would repress them to keep them hidden from awareness. These repressed experiences and feelings travel from the conscious mind location into the subconscious and unconscious mind. Although repressed and far from awareness, these feelings, thoughts, urges, and experiences could still affect and influence our behavior and decisions. Repressed thoughts and experiences are subliminally available to the conscious mind. They can show up in a series of thoughts, images, and sensations occurring in a person's mind during sleep. This is what we know as a dream. This is why Freud strongly believed that dream interpretation and analysis can help people learn what is going on within their unconscious thereby finding how those events influence their conscious actions. Our conscious mind interacts with our physical environment through speech, silence, change of position, and other physical actions. It interacts with our inward being through thoughts, fantasy, and other imaginary and imaginative impressions.

People often assume that all event processing occurs in the conscious mind. While your thinking and logical reasoning undoubtedly happen within the realm of the conscious mind, your unconscious mind is also adept at reasoning and logic. The human unconscious mind serves as a storage place for all memories, feelings, and habits.

THE METAMORPHOSIS OF THE MIND

When my second daughter was eighteen months old. She is a baby and I have observed critically her responses and learning curve. Her conscious mind had not yet developed fully enough to reason as an adult would. She cannot test, measure, and interpret all the information around her. What is currently going on within her less developed mind at this age is that her conscious mind is sitting in the background developing and building the capacity for information processing while her subconscious and unconscious performs all the data gathering and reasoning. She can identify my face and her mom's face. She can identify nipples as a source of food and express herself by crying. She observes our responses to her cry and uses that to develop her conscious mind. The subconscious and unconscious are the bedrock for the formation of conscious logical patterns that lead to a fully developed consciousness. Emotions, beliefs, and habits are the outcome of formed logical patterns with various events within the subconscious and unconscious mind of a growing child that could become a lifestyle in adulthood.

The human conscious mind represents the pinnacle of cognitive awareness, encompassing the immediate and deliberate aspects of thought. It is the realm of our waking awareness, where perceptions, thoughts, and experiences come into sharp focus. This facet of the mind enables individuals to engage with the external world, process information, and actively participate in decision-making.

Key characteristics of the human conscious mind include:
The conscious mind processes information in real time, allowing individuals to perceive their surroundings, interpret stimuli, and respond to the present moment.

Unlike the subconscious and unconscious aspects of the mind, the conscious mind is uniquely self-reflective. It enables individuals to recognize their thoughts, emotions, and actions, fostering a sense of self-awareness.

The ability to reflect on one's thoughts and experiences is a unique trait of the conscious mind. This capacity for introspection enables individuals to analyze and comprehend their internal states.

Conscious thought plays a central role in decision-making. Individuals can actively deliberate, weigh options, and make voluntary choices based on their conscious awareness and rational reasoning. The conscious mind is associated with logical thinking and reasoning abilities. It allows individuals to analyze information, solve problems, and engage in critical thinking processes.

The conscious mind is acutely aware of the passage of time. It allows individuals to perceive the sequential nature of events and maintain a continuous sense of the past, present, and future.

In summary, the human conscious mind is at the forefront of cognitive functioning, providing individuals with immediate awareness, self-reflection, and the capacity for deliberate thought and decision-making. It serves as the gateway to the external world and plays a crucial role in shaping our conscious experience.

Chapter 5

The Essence of Unconscious Mind

The unconscious mind refers to the part of our mental process that operates outside of our conscious awareness. This includes unconscious thoughts, feelings, and behaviors that are stored in our memory and influence our thoughts, emotions, and actions even though we may not be aware of them.

For example, our unconscious beliefs about ourselves and others, as well as our past experiences, can impact our current thoughts and behaviors. This can be seen in cases where a person has a strong emotional reaction to a certain situation, even though they are not consciously aware of why they are feeling this way.

The unconscious mind is also thought to play a crucial role in the formation of habits and automatic processes, such as driving a car or typing on a keyboard. These unconscious processes become so ingrained in our memory that they can be performed without conscious thought or effort.

Although the unconscious mind operates beyond our conscious awareness, it's not inaccessible or separate from our conscious mind. Techniques such as hypnosis, meditation, and psychotherapy can help bring unconscious thoughts and feelings to the surface, allowing individuals to gain greater insight and understanding of their unconscious mind and how it influences their lives.

The unconscious mind can also play a role in our decision-making processes. Research has shown that unconscious biases can influence our decisions and actions, even when we are not aware of them. For instance, studies have demonstrated that implicit biases can affect the hiring process, leading to discrimination against certain groups. In such cases, individuals may not be aware of these biases, but they still impact their actions and decisions.

The unconscious mind can also play a role in the development of mental health conditions such as anxiety and depression. Traumatic experiences or negative beliefs and experiences can be stored in the unconscious mind and influence our thoughts, behaviors, and emotions.

The unconscious mind is constantly processing information, even when we are not consciously aware of it. This means that our unconscious mind is constantly learning and adapting to new information and experiences.

Key aspects of the human unconscious mind include:
The unconscious mind encompasses mental processes that occur outside the sphere of conscious awareness. It holds thoughts, emotions, and memories that may be hidden from immediate introspection.

Many functions of the unconscious mind are automatic and instinctual. This includes processes such as breathing, heartbeat regulation, and reflex actions, which happen without conscious control.

The unconscious mind stores implicit memories—memories that influence behavior and responses without conscious recall. These memories may be associated with past experiences, conditioning, or learned behaviors. The unconscious often communicates through symbols, dreams, and metaphors. It expresses aspects of the psyche that may not be readily articulated in conscious thought.

The unconscious mind plays a role in defense mechanisms that protect the individual from overwhelming emotions or threatening thoughts. This includes mechanisms like repression, denial, and projection.

Emotions held in the unconscious mind can impact daily experiences and reactions. Unacknowledged feelings may surface in subtle ways, affecting mood, relationships, and decision-making.

The unconscious mind is considered a wellspring of creativity. It can generate novel ideas, insights, and solutions that may not be immediately apparent in conscious thought.

Understanding the human unconscious mind involves exploring these hidden dimensions and acknowledging the profound impact it exerts on behavior and psychological well-being. While the conscious mind operates in the light of awareness, the unconscious mind operates in the shadows, shaping the complexity of human experience in ways that often require exploration and interpretation.

THE METAMORPHOSIS OF THE MIND

Chapter 6

The District of Subconscious Mind

The subconscious mind refers to the part of the mind that is responsible for processing information that is below the level of conscious awareness. Unlike the conscious mind, which is responsible for our thoughts, perceptions, and decisions that we are aware of, the subconscious mind operates at a deeper level, outside of our conscious awareness.

Some of the functions of the subconscious mind include regulating our habits, automatic thoughts, and behaviors, and influencing our emotions. It also plays a role in storing and retrieving memories, as well as processing information about the world around us and guiding our behavior based on that information.

For example, if an individual learns to associate a specific sound with fear (e.g., hearing a car backfire), the subconscious mind may automatically respond with fear in the future whenever that sound is heard, even if the individual is not consciously aware of the fear response.

The subconscious mind can also impact our beliefs and attitudes. For example, if an individual grows up hearing negative messages about themselves, such as "you're not smart enough," those negative beliefs can become deeply ingrained in the subconscious mind and impact their self-esteem and confidence in the future.

The subconscious mind is a powerful and influential part of our mental processes. Understanding its role and impact can help individuals take steps to cultivate positive beliefs, attitudes, and behaviors.

In terms of psychology and therapy, the subconscious mind is often considered to be a rich source of insight and information about an individual's thoughts, feelings, and behaviors. Some therapeutic approaches, such as hypnotherapy and psychoanalytic therapy, aim to access the subconscious mind to uncover unconscious thoughts, beliefs, and emotions that may be contributing to psychological distress or impeding personal growth.

The subconscious mind, often likened to a silent orchestrator behind the scenes, serves as a vital bridge connecting the conscious and unconscious realms of human cognition. Within this bridge, intricate blueprints are stored—blueprints that chart the course of ingrained habits, learned behaviors, and the rich nature of our narrative.

Imagine the morning routine of brewing coffee or reaching for a phone upon waking. These actions, seemingly automatic, are manifestations of deeply ingrained habits residing within the subconscious. The subconscious mind stores the repetitive sequences of behavior, enabling individuals to carry out daily tasks with efficiency and minimal conscious effort.

THE METAMORPHOSIS OF THE MIND

As we go through life, we experience various situations that influence how we respond and behave. The subconscious mind serves as a repository for these learned behaviors, storing the lessons acquired from past experiences. For instance, a person who has learned to navigate social interactions through observation and experience may find their subconscious guiding them in social settings without conscious deliberation.

Our narrative, the story we tell ourselves about who we are, finds its threads woven within the subconscious mind. From childhood memories to significant life events, the subconscious holds the elements that contribute to the narrative shaping our identity. For example, an individual who associates success with hard work may find this belief rooted in the subconscious, influencing their approach to professional endeavors.

In moments of stress or danger, the subconscious mind swiftly triggers automatic responses, such as the fight-or-flight reaction. These responses are finely tuned blueprints designed to ensure survival. An individual experiencing heightened alertness during a perceived threat is, in essence, guided by the subconscious mind's intricate coding for self-preservation.

Cultural influences and societal norms become ingrained within the subconscious, shaping beliefs and influencing behavior. For instance, an individual raised in a culture valuing humility may find their subconscious guiding them towards modest actions, even in the absence of conscious thought.

Understanding the subconscious mind as a bridge provides a lens through which we can unravel the intricacies of our actions, reactions, and the narratives that shape our lives. It is within this bridge that the blueprints of our habits, learned behaviors, and personal stories are meticulously stored, influencing the nature of our existence.

Key features of the human subconscious mind include:
The subconscious mind serves as a repository for information and experiences that, while not in the forefront of awareness, can be readily accessed. This includes learned skills, past events, and cultural conditioning.

Patterns of behavior, habits, and reactions often originate from the subconscious. These automatic responses are shaped by past experiences and can impact daily actions without the individual consciously deliberating.

The subconscious mind excels in recognizing patterns and making connections. It aids in the interpretation of situations by drawing on stored knowledge, allowing for quick assessments and responses.

Emotions held in the subconscious mind can influence mood and reactions. Unresolved emotions or experiences may surface in response to stimuli, affecting overall emotional well-being.

The subconscious mind is instrumental in the process of learning and conditioning. It absorbs information from the environment, forms associations, and adapts behavior based on past experiences.

Like the unconscious mind, the subconscious contributes to creativity. It generates ideas, insights, and solutions by drawing on a vast reservoir of information, often presenting novel perspectives to the conscious mind.

During the dream state, the subconscious mind becomes more prominent. Dreams can be seen as a symbolic expression of the subconscious, offering glimpses into unprocessed emotions, desires, or unresolved issues.

Understanding the human subconscious mind involves recognizing its role as a dynamic intermediary that bridges conscious awareness and deeper unconscious processes. By exploring and acknowledging the influence of the subconscious, individuals gain insight into the layers of their cognitive and emotional landscape, paving the way for personal growth and self-awareness.

The subconscious mind is a complex and important aspect of the mind that plays a major role in shaping our thoughts, behaviors, and emotions. Understanding the power of the subconscious mind and taking steps to influence it in positive ways can have a significant impact on our overall well-being and quality of life.

In essence, "The Tripartite Nature of the Mind" beckons us to perceive the mind not as a singular entity but as a dynamic triad of conscious awareness, hidden depths, and the silent orchestrations of the subconscious. Together, these dimensions create a harmonious symphony, shaping the kaleidoscope of human experience and paving the way for a deeper understanding of the intricacies that define our cognitive existence.

THE METAMORPHOSIS OF THE MIND

Chapter 7

The Five Powers of the Mind

1. The power of perception
The power of perception refers to the process by which individuals construct meaning from sensory information that they receive from the world around them. In the context of the human mind, perception is how people interpret, organize, and make sense of information to understand their environment and make decisions.

The way that people perceive things is influenced by several factors, including past experiences, cultural background, beliefs, and emotions. The power of perception plays a critical role in shaping individuals' thoughts, behaviors, and decisions. For example, if someone has a negative perception of a particular person, they may avoid that person or treat them poorly, whereas if someone has a positive perception of that same person, they may be more likely to form a close relationship.

In short, the power of perception can greatly impact how people see the world and how they respond to it. By being aware of how perception works and how it influences their thoughts and behaviors, individuals can work to change their perceptions and create a more positive and fulfilling life.

Perception refers to how individuals interpret and make sense of sensory information from their environment. It influences our beliefs, attitudes, and actions. Our perception is shaped by our past experiences, emotions, expectations, cultural background, and other factors. The power of perception is the idea that our perceptions have a strong impact on our thoughts, feelings, and behavior.

For example, if a person perceives a situation as dangerous, they will feel anxious and may try to avoid the perceived danger. On the other hand, if a person perceives the same situation as an opportunity, they will feel more positive and confident, and be more likely to take action. Our perception has a major impact on how we experience the world and our place in it.

Therefore, it is important to be mindful of our perceptions and how they shape our experiences, and to make an effort to broaden our perspective and challenge negative perceptions. This can lead to a more positive and fulfilling life.

Our perception often operates with the principle of association. This is especially the case when they are not an import from our intuition. The principle of association implies that our thoughts, feelings, and behaviors are connected through associative links. For example, the smell of freshly baked cookies may bring back happy memories from childhood.

Association reveals that information in the mind is connected and stored in an interconnected network of memories, thoughts, and ideas. This means that the mind links new information with existing memories and knowledge, creating connections and associations between them.

For example, if you associate the smell of freshly baked cookies with happy memories from your childhood, the smell of cookies will trigger positive emotions and memories every time you encounter them. This is why the smell of certain foods, scents, or sounds can evoke strong emotions and memories.

Association also has implications for how we learn and remember information. Research has shown that information that is associated with meaningful, relevant, or emotionally charged information is more likely to be remembered, whereas information that is presented in an isolated or arbitrary manner is less likely to be retained. This is why it is often helpful to make connections between new information and our existing knowledge and experiences, such as creating mnemonics or linking new information to personal interests or values.

Furthermore, an association can also influence our thoughts and emotions. When we associate negative experiences or emotions with certain situations or individuals, we are more likely to experience similar emotions in the future when we encounter those situations or individuals again. This is why it is important to be mindful of the associations we create, and to make an effort to disassociate from negative experiences and emotions and associate with positive ones.

Association is a crucial principle of the human mind that has important implications for our ability to learn, remember, and experience information. By understanding this principle, we can create meaningful connections between new information and our existing knowledge, use mnemonics and other strategies to improve memory and cultivate positive associations and emotions to enhance our overall well-being.

Additionally, association highlights the importance of context in shaping our memories and experiences. The context in which information is encountered can greatly influence how it is processed, stored, and retrieved in the future. For example, memories of a particular event are often stronger when they are formed in a unique or unusual context, such as a particularly memorable location, or during an emotionally charged moment.

The association also plays a critical role in the formation of habits and automatic behaviors. Habits are formed through repeated associations between a particular behavior and a specific context, such as the habit of brushing your teeth every morning after waking up. As these associations become stronger over time, the behavior becomes automatic and requires little conscious effort to perform.

Moreover, an association has implications for creativity and problem-solving. By connecting new information with existing knowledge and experiences, we can form new insights, ideas, and solutions that would not have been possible without these connections. This is why it is often helpful to approach new problems from different perspectives, make connections with diverse experiences, and draw upon a wide range of knowledge and experiences to solve problems more effectively.

In conclusion, association is a fundamental principle of the human mind that plays a critical role in shaping our memories, habits, emotions, and problem-solving abilities. By understanding this principle, we can leverage its power to improve our ability to learn, remember, and experience information, as well as enhance our creativity and problem-solving skills.

2. The power of introspection/inclination
Introspection refers to the examination of one's thoughts, feelings, and emotions. It is the process of looking inward, self-observing, and self-reflection. The power of introspection refers to the capacity of an individual to understand their own mental and emotional states and to be aware of the impact they have on one's thoughts, feelings, and behaviors.

Introspection is powerful because it helps individuals understand their minds and behavior, allowing them to identify and change negative patterns and habits. For example, if an individual has a habit of overthinking and constantly worrying, introspection can help them understand the root causes of these behaviors and work to change them.

Introspection can also help individuals identify and understand their strengths and weaknesses, leading to greater self-awareness and personal growth. Additionally, it allows individuals to reflect on their experiences, feelings, and thoughts, leading to deeper self-understanding and a better understanding of the world around them.

Overall, the power of introspection is a valuable resource for individuals seeking to improve their mental and emotional well-being and to live a more fulfilling life.

Introspection refers to the act of reflecting on one's thoughts, emotions, and experiences. This process allows individuals to gain a deeper understanding of their own mental processes and inner workings. Through introspection, people can examine their thoughts and feelings objectively, identify patterns, and make changes to improve their mental health and well-being.

The power of introspection is significant in that it provides individuals with an opportunity to gain insight into their minds and thoughts. This type of self-reflection can lead to increased self-awareness and better decision-making, as well as improved mental health and well-being. Additionally, introspection can provide individuals with a deeper understanding of the underlying causes of their emotions and behaviors, allowing them to work towards resolving any issues they may be facing.

However, being completely honest with oneself and confronting negative thoughts and feelings can be difficult. Some may find introspection challenging due to a lack of experience or difficulty accessing inner thoughts and feelings.

Overall, the power of introspection is a valuable tool for individuals seeking to improve their mental health and well-being, and for those looking to gain a deeper understanding of their thoughts, emotions, and experiences.

3. The power of reflection
The power of reflection refers to the ability of the human mind to engage in self-reflection, introspection, and contemplation. It is the process of examining one's thoughts, emotions, beliefs, and actions

to gain a greater understanding of oneself and to make changes in behavior and attitudes.

Reflection enables individuals to evaluate their experiences, thoughts, and beliefs and make conscious choices about how they think and behave. It allows individuals to examine their assumptions, biases, and perspectives and to identify areas where they can make changes to improve their lives. Reflection can help individuals to develop greater self-awareness and to understand how their thoughts and emotions influence their experiences.

Reflection also plays an important role in learning and personal growth. By reflecting on past experiences and considering what worked well and what did not, individuals can gain new insights and develop new strategies for approaching challenges and opportunities.

Overall, the power of reflection allows individuals to become more intentional about their thoughts and behaviors, leading to greater self-awareness, personal growth, and overall well-being.

Reflection is the process of considering one's thoughts, feelings, and experiences and using that information to gain a deeper understanding of oneself and one's place in the world. This type of self-reflection can help people make positive changes in their lives and improve their mental health and well-being. Reflection can be thought of as a form of introspection, as it requires a person to look inward to gain insights into their thoughts and experiences.

Reflection can take many forms, including journaling, meditating, prayer, talking with a therapist or trusted friend, or simply taking time to be quiet and reflect on one's experiences and thoughts. It is important to set aside dedicated time for reflection, as this can help people develop a more intentional and mindful approach to life. Reflection can help individuals recognize patterns in their thoughts and behavior and identify areas where they may need to make changes.

There are many benefits of reflecting on one's thoughts and experiences, including improved emotional regulation, better relationships, and a greater sense of purpose and direction in life. Reflection can also help people identify their strengths and weaknesses and develop strategies for coping with stress and adversity. Reflection can also help people develop a greater appreciation for their experiences and an enhanced sense of gratitude and well-being.

In conclusion, the power of reflection is an important aspect of the human mind, as it allows people to gain a deeper understanding of themselves and their place in the world. Reflection can lead to improved mental health, greater self-awareness, and a more fulfilling life.

4. The power of retrospection
The power of retrospection refers to the ability of the human mind to recall past events and experiences. It involves looking back in time to reflect on past events and consider how they have shaped who we are and what we have learned from them. This ability allows us to examine our past behavior and make changes in the present or future to improve our lives and well-being. The power of retrospection is a valuable tool in self-reflection and personal growth as it allows us to gain insights into our patterns of behavior

and thought and identify areas for improvement. By reflecting on our past experiences and what we have learned from them, we can gain a deeper understanding of our motivations, beliefs, and emotions, and develop a stronger sense of self-awareness.

The power of retrospection refers to the ability of the human mind to reflect on past experiences, events, and emotions. It involves revisiting memories and considering how they have influenced one's thoughts, behaviors, and emotions. This ability allows individuals to gain a deeper understanding of themselves and to identify patterns and habits that may be holding them back.

Retrospection can also help individuals gain insight into past decisions and the thought processes that led to them. By reflecting on the past, individuals can gain a clearer understanding of their motivations, values, and beliefs, and make more informed decisions in the future. This can lead to personal growth and increased self-awareness.

In some cases, the power of retrospection can also have negative effects, such as causing feelings of regret, guilt, or self-blame. However, when used constructively, retrospection can help individuals improve their decision-making and promote positive change.

It is important to note that the power of retrospection is not limited to the conscious mind, as unconscious and subconscious processes can also play a role in shaping our thoughts and behaviors. As a result, individuals may not be aware of the full impact that past experiences have had on their lives, and engaging in regular retrospection can help them gain a deeper understanding of these influences.

Retrospection refers to the ability of a person to reflect on past experiences, memories, and emotions. This power is a crucial aspect of the human mind and allows individuals to gain insights and understanding from past experiences. It enables people to evaluate their past actions, thoughts, and behaviors, and to make necessary changes in the present and future. Retrospection is a valuable tool for personal growth, learning, and decision-making.

Retrospection is closely tied to the human mind, as it's through the mind that we recall and reflect on past experiences. This power allows us to bring forth memories and emotions from the past, and to analyze them in the present moment. Through retrospection, we can identify patterns of behavior and thought that have been hindering our progress and well-being. It allows us to understand our experiences more deeply, and to make positive changes to our lives.

Retrospection also helps us to gain a deeper understanding of our values and priorities, as well as to develop a clearer sense of purpose. This power can be a powerful tool for self-awareness and self-improvement and can lead to greater happiness and fulfillment in life. However, it is important to be mindful of the way we reflect on our past experiences, as it can also be easy to get stuck in negative thoughts and emotions. It is important to approach retrospection with an open mind and to focus on the positive aspects of our experiences.

The human mind can operate under the principle of Reversibility. This implies that the mind can operate in both forward and backward directions, meaning that we can both recall memories from the past and imagine potential scenarios and events in the future.

This has important implications for our ability to plan, make decisions, and evaluate potential outcomes. By imagining potential future scenarios, we can consider different courses of action and make informed decisions about the best path forward. Similarly, by recalling past experiences, we can reflect on our experiences and make more informed decisions in the present and future.

The principle of reversibility also highlights the importance of mental rehearsal, which refers to the process of practicing a particular behavior or scenario in the mind, as a way to prepare for future events. Research has shown that mental rehearsal can be a powerful tool for enhancing performance, improving confidence, and reducing stress and anxiety in performance situations.

Moreover, reversibility is also related to our ability to process and learn from experiences. By reflecting on past experiences and considering different scenarios, we can gain new insights, build new knowledge, and develop new skills and abilities.

The principle of reversibility is a critical principle of the human mind that plays a key role in our ability to imagine, plan, reflect, and learn from experiences. By understanding and applying this principle, we can harness the power of our imagination to make more informed decisions, improve performance, and enhance our ability to process and learn from experiences.

Furthermore, reversibility also highlights the power of visualization and positive affirmations in shaping our thoughts, emotions, and actions. By visualizing positive outcomes and repeating positive affirmations, we can influence our subconscious mind to act in ways that are aligned with our goals and aspirations.

For example, athletes often use visualization techniques to mentally rehearse their performance before a competition, imagining themselves executing their skills with precision and confidence. Similarly, individuals who wish to overcome negative thoughts or emotions can use affirmations and visualization to replace those thoughts with more positive and empowering ones.

In addition, reversibility also has implications for our mental and emotional well-being. By recalling positive experiences and imagining positive scenarios, we can increase feelings of happiness and positivity, whereas recalling negative experiences and imagining negative scenarios can increase feelings of anxiety and depression. This is why it is important to be mindful of the thoughts and images we allow into our minds, making an effort to focus on positive and empowering ones.

In conclusion, the principle of reversibility highlights the power of the human mind to imagine, recall, and process information in both forward and backward directions. By understanding and applying this principle, we can use visualization, positive affirmations, and reflective practices to improve our mental and emotional well-being, enhance our performance, and shape our thoughts and actions in positive ways.

5. The power of human imagination

The imagination is the life wire that links the mind to the brain. The heart ensures that the entire cell, tissue, organ, and systems of the human body are constantly fed with oxygenated blood as deoxygenated blood is returned to it to be oxygenated. The mind ensures that the will, emotion, and memory are fed with general or specialized knowledge at every point in time whereas unexplainable events and issues are extracted from them and handed to the mind for explanation and generation of the required answers. In the Bible, the heart and the mind are interchangeable either for translational reasons or because certain words can be used for two or more related things. The mind is used for the heart as the heart for the mind. But by contextual understanding, one can distinguish one to be the physical heart and the other to belong to the soulish realm.

The imagination is the lens that magnifies and reveals details or content of a thing. It passes the information through the thought-line for further development or a long-range view. Thou wilt keep him perfect peace, whose mind is stayed on thee: because he trusteth in thee" (Isa. 26:3).

The thought or imagination is the instrument for meditation. During meditation, imagination is employed to press continually on the intuition, objective, and creative imagination for infinite knowledge applicable to problem-solving and understanding of a thing. A troubled and confused mind can receive quietness and joy when its thought and imagination are focused on God for true knowledge and revelation. Peace of mind is a function of clarity and enlightenment from the Spirit of God which empowers and fills the mind with pure thought and imagination.

The power of human imagination refers to our ability to conceive of and create mental images, scenarios, and ideas that are not limited by our current reality. It allows us to explore and envision new possibilities, invent new things, and solve problems in creative ways.

For example, the power of human imagination led to the creation of works of art, literature, and music that have captured the hearts and minds of people for centuries. It also gave rise to technological advancements such as flight, computers, and the internet, as well as scientific discoveries such as theories of evolution and quantum mechanics.

Creativity is the child of human imagination. It is the idea that the human mind has the innate ability to create and conceive new ideas, concepts, and solutions. This principle of creativity and conception refers to the ability of the mind to generate original and innovative thoughts through the process of combining and recombining existing information in new and imaginative ways.

Creativity and conception are vital components of human progress and innovation, and they play an important role in many fields, including science, art, technology, and entrepreneurship. The human mind can visualize new possibilities, imagine new worlds and new ways of doing things, and bring these ideas to life.

This principle of creativity and conception is based on the idea that the human mind is an active participant in shaping its own experiences and the world around it. Our thoughts and beliefs can influence our perceptions, and our perceptions can shape our reality.

Research has shown that the ability to be creative and conceive new ideas can be enhanced through a variety of practices, including mindfulness, brainstorming, and other forms of divergent thinking. Additionally, embracing a growth mindset, where individuals believe their abilities can be developed through effort and experience, has been shown to foster creative thinking and problem-solving skills.

Creativity and conception highlight the power of the human mind to generate new ideas and bring them to life. By embracing creativity and embracing a growth mindset, individuals can tap into their innate ability to conceive and bring new ideas to the world, driving progress and innovation in all areas of life.

Furthermore, creativity and conception highlight the importance of creating an environment that fosters creativity and innovation. This may involve encouraging experimentation and risk-taking, providing opportunities for collaboration and idea-sharing, and promoting a culture of continuous learning and growth.

In addition, it is also important to recognize that the process of creativity and conception is not always linear and may involve failures, setbacks, and moments of frustration. However, it is important to embrace the idea of trial and error and to view these experiences as opportunities to learn, grow, and refine one's creative abilities.

Moreover, creativity and conception also underscore the importance of recognizing and valuing the creative contributions of individuals, regardless of their background, education, or experience. Encouraging diversity of thought and valuing a range of perspectives can lead to a more dynamic and innovative environment, where new ideas and perspectives are more likely to emerge and thrive.

Creativity and conception also highlight the essential role that creativity and innovation play in driving progress and growth in all areas of life. By fostering an environment that nurtures creativity, valuing the contributions of diverse individuals, and embracing a growth mindset, individuals and organizations can tap into their full potential for creativity and innovation.

In everyday life, the power of imagination allows individuals to dream of a better future, imagine alternative solutions to problems, and create new ideas that have the potential to change the world. It is a fundamental aspect of human nature and can inspire and transform the way we live and interact with each other.

The power of human imagination is a remarkable and unique ability that sets us apart from other species. It is an innate capacity that allows us to create mental images, scenarios, and ideas that do not necessarily exist in our physical world. The power of imagination is not limited by the laws of nature, time, or space and can be used to explore a limitless range of possibilities and perspectives.

Imagination can take many forms, including visualizing new ideas, concepts, and inventions; dreaming up alternative solutions to problems; and creating works of art, literature, music, and other forms of cultural expression. It also plays a crucial role in scientific discovery, as scientists and researchers use their imaginations to develop new theories, hypotheses, and experiments that push the boundaries of our understanding of the world.

The power of human imagination is not just limited to the arts and sciences, however. It is also a critical component of our everyday lives. By using our imaginations, we can dream of a better future, envision alternative outcomes to difficult situations, and find new and innovative ways to tackle everyday challenges.

A vivid and imaginative story can stir our emotions and transport us to another world, while the power of imagination can also help us process and cope with difficult emotions and experiences.

The power of human imagination is a remarkable and essential aspect of our humanity. It allows us to explore and create new ideas, to imagine alternative solutions to problems, and to experience a wide range of emotions and perspectives. It is a powerful tool that can inspire and transform the world in which we live.

The power of human imagination is not just limited to the individual level but also has significant societal and cultural implications. It has been used throughout history to challenge prevailing ideas and beliefs, to promote social change, and to bring about political and economic transformation.

For example, movements such as the civil rights movement and the fight for gender equality were driven by individuals who used their imaginations to envision a world where everyone was treated with equality and respect. These movements challenged the dominant beliefs of their time and helped to bring about significant social change.

Similarly, the imagination has been used to promote economic development and growth. Entrepreneurs and innovators use their imaginations to conceive new products, services, and business models that have the potential to revolutionize industries and create new forms of wealth and prosperity.

In short, the power of human imagination is a powerful force for good in the world. It allows us to envision new possibilities, challenge prevailing ideas and beliefs, and promote positive change on both the individual and societal levels. It is a critical component of our humanity and an essential tool for shaping a better future.

The ability to imagine, dream, and create is truly a gift and it is up to each individual to harness this power and use it to make a positive impact on the world. Whether it is through art, science, business, or social activism, the power of human imagination has the potential to inspire and transform the world in profound ways.

It is important to note that the power of imagination is not just limited to conscious, deliberate acts of creation, but also extends to our subconscious and spontaneous thoughts. The human mind is constantly generating new ideas and images, whether we are aware of it or not.

In some cases, these spontaneous imaginations can lead to unexpected insights and breakthroughs. For example, a person might have a sudden epiphany while taking a shower or going for a walk, revealing a solution to a problem that had previously seemed unsolvable. This is because the mind is free to explore and connect ideas and concepts in new and innovative ways when it is not constrained by conscious thought.

Moreover, imagination can also be cultivated and developed through intentional effort and practice. People who are highly imaginative and creative tend to have a rich inner world, constantly generating new ideas and experimenting with different perspectives. They also tend to have a strong curiosity and a willingness to take risks and explore new possibilities.

In conclusion, the power of human imagination is a multifaceted and complex ability that has the potential to change our lives and the world in profound ways. It is a powerful tool that can be harnessed and developed through intentional effort and practice, allowing us to imagine and create a better future. Whether it is through conscious creation or spontaneous thought, the power of human imagination is a gift that should be cherished and cultivated.

THE METAMORPHOSIS OF THE MIND

Chapter 8

The Five Laws of the Mind

There is no widely accepted set of "laws" of the human mind, but some principles that are widely recognized in the field of psychology and neuroscience include:

It is important to note that these principles are not absolute laws and are not applicable in every situation. However, they provide a useful framework for understanding some of the fundamental processes of the human mind.

It is also worth mentioning that these principles are not exhaustive and many other factors influence the functioning of the human mind. For example, the effects of past experiences, social and cultural influences, and individual differences in personality, motivation, and cognitive style can also have a significant impact on the workings of the human mind.

Additionally, these principles are not static and can change over time. As we gain new experiences, learn new information, and engage in new activities, our thoughts, behaviors, and emotions are continually shaped and molded by the ongoing processes of the human mind.

Furthermore, these principles are also interconnected and can interact with each other in complex ways. For example, the emotions we experience can influence the information we attend to and the decisions we make, and our attention can be shaped by our goals, values, and the relevance of information to our current needs.

The five laws of the human mind provide a useful framework for understanding some of the fundamental processes of the human mind. However, these principles are subject to change and influence by a multitude of factors. A deeper understanding of the workings of the human mind requires a comprehensive and multidisciplinary approach that considers the complex interplay of biological, psychological, and social factors.

1. The Law of Attention:
This principle states that the mind can only focus on a limited amount of information at any given time. The more attention we give to something, the more it becomes ingrained in our memory and the more influence it has on our thoughts and behaviors.

The Law of Attention states that the mind can only focus on a limited amount of information at any given time. This means that the mind has a limited capacity to process and retain information, and it must prioritize which information to attend to and which to ignore. The principle of attention is closely related to the concept of cognitive load, which refers to the amount of mental effort required to process information. When the cognitive load becomes too great, the mind becomes overwhelmed and is less able to process and retain information effectively.

The law of attention also has implications for how we learn and remember information. Research has shown that information that is given our full attention is more likely to be remembered, whereas information that is only passively processed is less likely to be retained. This is why it is important to be fully present and engaged when learning new information and to take breaks when we need to refocus our attention.

Moreover, the law of attention can also influence our perception and interpretation of the world around us. When our attention is focused on one particular aspect of a situation, we are more likely to overlook other important details, and our perceptions and interpretations of the situation can be shaped by our attentional focus.

In conclusion, the law of attention is a crucial principle of the human mind that has important implications for our ability to process, retain, and interpret information. By understanding this principle, we can develop strategies to maximize our attentional capacity, such as taking breaks when our attention becomes overwhelmed, focusing our attention when learning new information, and being mindful of our attentional focus when interpreting the world around us.

Additionally, the law of attention has implications for our mental health and well-being. Research has shown that our attentional capacity can be affected by stress, anxiety, and other forms of emotional distress, leading to difficulties in focusing and retaining information. In these cases, it can be helpful to engage in stress-reduction techniques such as mindfulness meditation, exercise, and deep breathing exercises to improve attentional capacity.

Another important aspect of the law of attention is that it is influenced by our goals and motivations. When we are motivated to achieve a specific goal, such as learning a new skill or completing a task, we are more likely to allocate our attentional resources towards that goal, enabling us to process and retain information more effectively.

Moreover, the law of attention also highlights the importance of mindful attention, which refers to the ability to focus our attention on the present moment and be fully engaged in our experiences. Mindful attention has been shown to improve attentional capacity, reduce stress and anxiety, and enhance overall well-being.

In conclusion, the law of attention is a critical principle of the human mind that has far-reaching implications for our ability to process and retain information, our mental health and well-being, and our ability to achieve our goals and live fulfilling lives. By understanding and applying the principles of the law of attention, we can improve our cognitive functioning and enhance our quality of life.

2. The Law of Repetition:
This principle states that the more often an idea or behavior is repeated, the more likely it is to become automatic and ingrained in our minds. This is why repetition is a key element of learning and memory.

The Law of Repetition states that repeated experiences and practices have a lasting impact on our thoughts, emotions, and behavior. This law highlights the power of repetition to shape our habits, beliefs, and values, as well as to form new neural connections in the brain.

For example, repeating a particular behavior regularly can turn it into a habit, and over time, the behavior can become automatic and unconscious. This is why it is easier to maintain a habit that we have been practicing for a long time compared to a new one we are just starting to develop.

The law of repetition also applies to our thoughts and beliefs, as repeated thoughts and experiences can shape our attitudes and values over time. For example, if we repeat positive affirmations or engage in positive visualization practices, we can influence our subconscious mind to adopt a more positive outlook, leading to an increase in confidence, motivation, and well-being.

In addition, the law of repetition has implications for learning and skill acquisition, as repeated exposure to new information and experiences can increase our understanding and mastery of the material. This is why repetition is often used as a key strategy in teaching and learning, as it helps consolidate new information and make it more easily accessible in the future.

The law of repetition highlights the power of repeated experiences and practices to shape our thoughts, emotions, and behavior over time. We can use repetition as a tool to develop new habits, cultivate positive thoughts and beliefs, and enhance our learning and skill acquisition.

Furthermore, the law of repetition is also relevant to our emotions, as repeated emotional experiences can shape our emotional responses over time. For example, repeated exposure to fear or stress can increase our level of anxiety and fearfulness, whereas repeated exposure to positive and enjoyable experiences can increase our level of happiness and well-being.

It is also worth noting that the law of repetition applies to negative experiences and behaviors as well. For example, repeating negative self-talk or engaging in self-destructive behaviors can have a lasting impact on our mental and emotional health. This is why it is important to be mindful of our thoughts, behaviors, and emotional responses, and to make an effort to repeat positive and constructive experiences and practices.

In conclusion, the law of repetition highlights the power of repeated experiences and practices to shape our thoughts, emotions, and behavior over time. By understanding and applying this principle, we can use repetition as a tool to cultivate positive and constructive experiences and practices and enhance our mental and emotional health.

3. The Law of Relevance:
This principle states that the mind is more likely to attend to and remember information that is perceived as relevant or important to our goals, needs, and values. Information that is perceived as irrelevant or unimportant is less likely to be processed and retained by the mind.

The Law of Relevance highlights the crucial role that relevance plays in shaping our perception and memory. Our mind is designed to prioritize information that is perceived as relevant or important to our goals, needs, and values, as this information is more likely to be relevant to our survival and success.

For example, if we are studying for an exam, information that is directly related to the exam topics is likely to be perceived as more relevant and important, and thus, more easily remembered. On the other hand, information that is perceived as irrelevant or unimportant is likely to be forgotten or ignored.

Moreover, the law of relevance is also relevant to our decision-making. When making decisions, we tend to consider information that is relevant or important to our goals, needs, and values, and disregard information that is perceived as irrelevant or unimportant. This is why it is important to understand our goals, needs, and values, as they help to guide our attention and decision-making.

Our feelings play a crucial role in shaping our thoughts, behaviors, and decision-making. Feelings serve as a powerful motivator and can override even our most rational thoughts and intentions. The power of our emotions can influence our perception of reality and drive our actions and decision-making. It tends to take the upper hand in terms of influencing our minds and our preferences.

For example, when we experience strong feelings such as fear, excitement, or joy, our thoughts and behavior are likely to be impacted. Fear, for instance, can cause us to become more cautious and avoidant, while excitement can increase our motivation and drive. Similarly, positive emotions such as joy and happiness can increase our well-being, creativity, and overall satisfaction with life.

Moreover, our feelings also shape our beliefs and attitudes over time. For instance, if we repeatedly experience positive emotions in a particular situation, we are likely to develop a positive attitude towards that situation, and vice versa. This is why it is important to cultivate positive emotions and avoid negative ones, as they can have a lasting impact on our mental and emotional health.

The power of feelings highlights the power of our emotions to shape our thoughts, beliefs, and behavior. By understanding and applying this principle, we can use our emotions as a tool to enhance our well-being, improve our decision-making, and cultivate positive attitudes and beliefs.

Additionally, the power of feelings also highlights the importance of emotional regulation and management. Our emotional responses are not always in our control, but we can learn to manage them in ways that are constructive and positive. For example, we can practice mindfulness and meditation to increase our emotional intelligence and resilience or engage in activities that bring us joy and happiness to cultivate positive emotions.

It is also important to understand that our feelings are interconnected and can influence each other. For instance, if we experience anger, it can trigger feelings of frustration, anxiety, and even depression. On the other hand, experiencing positive emotions such as gratitude and love can enhance our sense of well-being and resilience.

The influence of feelings highlights the power of our emotions to shape our thoughts, beliefs, and behavior. We can use our emotions as a tool to enhance our well-being, improve our decision-making, and cultivate positive attitudes and beliefs. By learning to regulate and manage our emotions, we can increase our emotional intelligence, resilience, and overall mental and emotional health.

The law of relevance highlights the importance of relevance in shaping our perception, memory, and decision-making. By understanding and applying this principle, we can use relevance as a tool to focus our attention and enhance our learning and decision-making. By prioritizing information that is relevant or important to our goals, needs, and values, we can increase our productivity, efficiency, and overall success in life.

Additionally, the law of relevance also highlights the importance of context in shaping our perception and memory. Our perception and memory of information can be greatly influenced by the context in which it is presented or experienced. For instance, information that is presented in a positive or neutral context is more likely to be perceived as relevant or important, while information that is presented in a negative or irrelevant context is more likely to be disregarded or forgotten.

This principle is also relevant to our decision-making, as context can influence our perception of the importance and relevance of information, and thus, our decisions. For example, if we are deciding on a job opportunity, information about the company culture, benefits, and work-life balance may be perceived as relevant and important, while information about the company's location or commute may be perceived as less relevant.

In conclusion, the law of relevance highlights the important role that relevance and context play in shaping our perception, memory, and decision-making. By understanding and applying this principle, we can use relevance and context as tools to focus our attention, enhance our learning, and improve our decision-making. By prioritizing the information that is relevant and important to our goals, needs, and values, and by considering the context in which information is presented, we can increase our productivity, efficiency, and overall success in life.

4. The law of belief
The law of belief refers to the idea that our beliefs and attitudes shape our perceptions and experiences of the world. This principle states that what we believe about ourselves, others, and the world around us has a powerful influence on our thoughts, feelings, and behaviors.

According to this law, our beliefs can act as self-fulfilling prophecies, shaping our perceptions and experiences in ways that align with our expectations. For example, if we believe that we are capable, we are more likely to approach challenges with confidence and resilience and to experience success as a result. Conversely, if we believe that we are inadequate or inferior, we may avoid challenges and experience failure and disappointment.

A multidimensional analysis across 21 countries revealed that well-being involves positive emotions, personal development, control over one's life, a sense of purpose, and positive relationships.[16] It is therefore important to be mindful of the beliefs and attitudes that shape our perceptions and experiences and to strive to adopt beliefs

---

[16] Well-being is more than happiness and life satisfaction: a multidimensional analysis of 21 countries | Health and Quality of Life Outcomes | Full Text (biomedcentral.com).

and attitudes that are supportive, empowering, and in alignment with our values and goals.

In addition, the law of belief also highlights the importance of being mindful of the beliefs and attitudes that are shaped by our culture, family, and other social institutions. It also emphasizes the impact these beliefs and attitudes can have on our perceptions and experiences.

The law of belief highlights the power of our beliefs and attitudes to shape our perceptions and experiences of the world. By being mindful of the beliefs and attitudes that influence our thoughts, feelings, and behaviors, and striving to adopt beliefs that are supportive, empowering, and in alignment with our values and goals, we can tap into the full potential of the law of belief and create a more fulfilling and fulfilling life.

Furthermore, the law of belief also acknowledges that beliefs can change and evolve, as we gain new experiences and insights, and that this process of change is an important aspect of personal growth and development. By being open-minded and receptive to new perspectives and experiences, individuals can expand their beliefs and attitudes, and develop a more nuanced and inclusive view of the world.

In addition, the law of belief also highlights the importance of considering the beliefs and attitudes of others and striving to understand and respect the perspectives and experiences of those who may hold different beliefs and attitudes than ourselves. This can help to foster more harmonious and collaborative relationships and promote a more inclusive and diverse society.

Moreover, the law of belief also underscores the importance of being aware of limiting beliefs and attitudes and taking steps to challenge and overcome these beliefs. For example, an individual who holds a limiting belief that they are not capable of pursuing their dream career may need to challenge this belief and adopt a more empowering and supportive belief that they have the skills, knowledge, and experience to succeed.

In conclusion, the law of belief is a powerful principle that highlights the impact that our beliefs and attitudes have on our perceptions and experiences of the world. By being mindful of the beliefs and attitudes that shape our thoughts, feelings, and behaviors, and striving to adopt beliefs that are supportive, empowering, and in alignment with our values and goals, we can tap into the full potential of the law of belief and create a more fulfilling and meaningful life.

5. The Law of Expectation

The Law of Expectancy/Faith states that our beliefs and expectations about a particular outcome can greatly influence the outcome itself. This law highlights the power of the mind to shape reality, as our beliefs and expectations can influence our thoughts, emotions, and actions, and ultimately determine the outcome of a particular situation.

For example, if we believe that we will be successful in a particular task or project, we are more likely to approach the task with confidence and take actions that are aligned with our goal. Conversely, if we believe that we will fail, we may approach the task with fear and doubt, leading to a self-fulfilling prophecy.

This law also highlights the importance of setting and pursuing goals, as having a clear and positive expectation of a desired outcome can motivate and inspire us to take action and overcome obstacles along the way. Research has shown that individuals who set and pursue goals are more likely to achieve success than those who do not and that having a clear and positive expectation of success can increase motivation, confidence, and resilience in the face of challenges and obstacles.

Moreover, the law of expectancy has implications for our relationships, as our expectations about others can shape our interactions and perceptions of them. For example, if we have positive expectations about someone, we are more likely to approach the relationship with an open and positive attitude, leading to a more positive and productive relationship. Conversely, if we have negative expectations about someone, we may approach the relationship with suspicion and negativity, leading to a negative and unproductive relationship.

The law of expectancy highlights the power of our beliefs and expectations to shape our thoughts, emotions, and actions, and ultimately determine the outcome of a particular situation. We can harness the power of positive thinking and goal setting to improve our performance, relationships, and overall well-being.

Furthermore, the law of expectancy can also play a role in our mental and emotional health. By having optimistic expectations, we can increase our resilience and ability to cope with stress and adversity. On the other hand, having pessimistic expectations can lead to feelings of anxiety and depression, as well as increase the likelihood of stress-related health problems.

It is also worth noting that our expectations are not just limited to our thoughts and beliefs about a particular outcome, but also extend to our perceptions and interpretations of information and experiences. For example, if we expect a particular experience to be negative, we are more likely to interpret it as negative, even if objectively it may not be. This is why it is important to be mindful of our expectations and to make an effort to cultivate positive and optimistic ones.

The law of expectancy highlights the power of our beliefs and expectations to shape our thoughts, emotions, and actions, as well as our perceptions and interpretations of experiences. By understanding and applying this principle, we can cultivate positive and optimistic expectations, increase our resilience and ability to cope with stress and adversity and improve our mental and emotional health.

This principle is also relevant to our decision-making, as our beliefs and expectations influence what we consider and the choices we make. For example, if we believe that we can achieve our goals, we are more likely to take action and persist in the face of challenges. On the other hand, if we have negative beliefs or self-doubt, we may be less likely to take action and give up more easily.

In conclusion, the law of expectancy highlights the power of our beliefs and expectations to shape our perceptions, experiences, and outcomes. We can use our beliefs and expectations as tools to shape our perceptions, experiences, and outcomes in positive ways. By cultivating positive beliefs and expectations, we can increase our motivation, persistence, and overall success in life.

THE METAMORPHOSIS OF THE MIND

Chapter 9

The Stimuli of the Human Mind

The human mind functions like a dynamic ecosystem, gaining vitality and strength through exposure to a diverse array of stimuli. This statement underscores the idea that akin to the flourishing diversity within an ecosystem, the mind thrives when subjected to a variety of enriching factors. This diversity serves as nourishment for cognitive capacities, promoting growth, adaptability, and overall mental well-being. The analogy emphasizes the significance of exposing the mind to a rich nature of experiences, challenges, and sources of inspiration for optimal cognitive health and resilience. From intellectual pursuits to sensory experiences, the following factors act as catalysts for stimulating the human mind:

Engaging in intellectual pursuits such as reading, solving puzzles, and exploring new ideas provides the mind with the necessary stimulation to foster curiosity, critical thinking, and a continuous hunger for knowledge. Utilizing technology for exploration, whether through virtual reality, online courses, or interactive applications, introduces novel ways of learning and problem-solving, fostering digital literacy and cognitive adaptability. Diversifying learning experiences, whether through formal education, workshops, or hands-on activities, keeps the mind agile and receptive to new information. Learning stimulates neural connections and promotes cognitive flexibility. Engaging in problem-solving challenges, whether through puzzles, games, or real-life scenarios, stimulates cognitive functions such as analysis, pattern recognition, and strategic thinking. These challenges promote mental agility. Embracing a mindset of lifelong learning ensures a constant influx of new information and ideas. Whether through formal education or self-directed learning, the pursuit of knowledge keeps the mind vibrant and receptive.

Engaging in creative endeavors, whether through the realms of art, music, writing, or any form of self-expression, serves as a potent catalyst for stimulating the imaginative faculties of the mind. This expansive realm of creativity is not merely an outlet for artistic pursuits; it is a dynamic force that nurtures cognitive functions, fostering innovation, problem-solving, and emotional intelligence.

Creativity is the wellspring of innovation, providing a fertile ground for generating novel ideas and groundbreaking concepts. When individuals immerse themselves in creative expression, they challenge conventional thinking patterns, opening pathways for innovative solutions to emerge. This process encourages a mindset that embraces novelty, originality, and the courage to explore uncharted territories of thought.

Participation in creative activities cultivates a mindset adept at problem-solving. The imaginative process inherent in creative expression nurtures the ability to approach challenges with flexibility and adaptability. Creative thinkers often excel at finding unconventional solutions, leveraging their capacity to think outside conventional boundaries.

The emotional depth embedded in creative expression nurtures emotional intelligence, enhancing one's ability to understand and navigate complex emotions, both within oneself and in others. Whether through the strokes of a paintbrush, the notes of a melody, or the words on a page, creative endeavors provide an outlet for processing and expressing emotions, fostering greater emotional resilience.

Participating in creative activities requires the mind to embrace ambiguity and engage in divergent thinking. This process enhances cognitive flexibility, allowing individuals to adapt to new information and approach challenges from multiple perspectives. Creative expression thus becomes a dynamic exercise that strengthens the mind's ability to navigate the complexities of an ever-evolving world.

In essence, creative expression becomes a dynamic force that propels the mind towards innovation, refined problem-solving skills, emotional intelligence, and cognitive flexibility. By embracing and fostering creative endeavors, individuals unlock the transformative power of their imaginative faculties, contributing to a more vibrant and resilient cognitive landscape.

Engaging in regular physical exercise extends benefits beyond the realm of physical well-being, actively stimulating the mind. This holistic approach to health recognizes the intricate connection between physical activity, nutrition, and cognitive function, fostering an environment that enhances mental clarity and cognitive performance.

Physical exercise serves as a dynamic catalyst for increased blood flow to the brain. As the body engages in activities that elevate the heart rate, circulation improves, delivering a rich supply of oxygen and nutrients to the brain. This heightened blood flow is instrumental in maintaining optimal brain health and supporting various cognitive functions.

The act of exercising triggers the release of neurotransmitters, the chemical messengers that facilitate communication between brain cells. These neurotransmitters, including serotonin, dopamine, and norepinephrine, play crucial roles in regulating mood, attention, and overall mental well-being. The positive impact of physical activity on neurotransmitter release contributes to a more balanced and resilient mental state.

Function: Regular physical activity has been linked to improved cognitive function across various domains. It positively influences memory, attention, and executive functions, promoting sharper mental acuity. This cognitive enhancement is attributed to the neurobiological changes induced by exercise, such as the formation of new neural connections and the release of growth factors that support brain health.

The combination of increased blood flow, neurotransmitter release, and enhanced cognitive function culminates in improved mental clarity and focus. Individuals who incorporate regular physical exercise into their routines often experience heightened alertness and concentration, contributing to overall mental sharpness and productivity.

Recognizing the symbiotic relationship between physical exercise and nutrition, this approach encompasses a well-rounded commitment to overall well-being. A balanced and nutrient-rich diet complements the benefits of exercise, providing the essential elements required for optimal brain function. This holistic synergy ensures a comprehensive approach to maintaining both physical and mental health.

In essence, physical exercise and nutrition form a dynamic duo that not only nurtures the body but also actively stimulates the mind. By understanding and embracing this interconnected relationship, individuals can harness the power of a healthy lifestyle to cultivate mental clarity, cognitive resilience, and holistic well-being.

Mindfulness practices, encompassing meditation and deep-breathing exercises, emerge as powerful tools for stimulating the mind, fostering relaxation, stress reduction, and enhanced focus. Rooted in ancient traditions, these practices offer a contemporary approach to nurturing a heightened state of awareness and promoting overall mental well-being.

Mindfulness practices serve as a sanctuary for the mind, providing a tranquil space for relaxation and stress reduction. Through meditation and intentional breathing, individuals engage in a purposeful journey inward, allowing the mind to release tension and unwind from the demands of daily life. This deliberate focus on the present moment becomes a refuge from the pressures of the external world.

The disciplined nature of mindfulness practices contributes to enhanced focus and concentration. As individuals engage in meditation, they train the mind to anchor itself in the present, steering away from the distractions that often lead to scattered attention. This honing of attentional skills cultivates a mental clarity that extends beyond the meditative session, positively impacting daily tasks and responsibilities.

At the core of mindfulness practices lies the cultivation of a heightened state of awareness. By intentionally directing attention to the present moment, individuals become attuned to their thoughts, emotions, and bodily sensations. This self-awareness becomes a powerful tool for navigating the complexities of the mind, fostering emotional intelligence and a deeper understanding of one's internal landscape.

Mindfulness practices contribute significantly to overall mental well-being. The intentional focus on the present moment creates a sense of calm and inner peace, even in the face of life's challenges. Regular engagement in these practices has been linked to reduced symptoms of anxiety and depression, highlighting their transformative impact on emotional resilience.

The beauty of mindfulness practices lies in their adaptability to daily routines. Whether incorporated into morning rituals, work breaks, or bedtime routines, these practices seamlessly integrate into various aspects of life. This accessibility empowers individuals to infuse moments of mindfulness into their daily existence, cultivating an ongoing sense of mental balance.

In essence, meditation and mindfulness practices offer a pathway to cultivating mindful awareness, relaxation, and enhanced mental focus. This intentional journey inward becomes a sanctuary for the mind, providing a holistic approach to nurturing mental well-being amid life's demands.

Meaningful social interactions and engaging conversations provide mental stimulation by exposing the mind to diverse perspectives, ideas, and social cues. Collaboration and communication contribute to cognitive growth. Exposure to new environments, cultures, and experiences through travel stimulates the mind by challenging preconceptions and expanding one's worldview. Novel experiences encourage adaptability and broaden cognitive horizons. Spending time in nature has restorative effects on the mind. The sights, sounds, and smells of the natural environment provide a sensory stimulus that promotes relaxation, creativity, and overall well-being.

The fusion of meaningful social interactions and immersive exposure to nature forms a dynamic synergy that actively stimulates the mind, fostering cognitive growth, adaptability, and overall well-being. This holistic approach recognizes the profound impact of both social connections and nature's embrace on the intricate workings of the human mind.

Meaningful social interactions serve as a potent source of mental stimulation. Engaging in conversations with others exposes the mind to diverse perspectives, ideas, and social cues. The exchange of thoughts, emotions, and experiences within a social context provides a rich nature of stimuli, actively contributing to cognitive growth and expanding one's mental horizons.

Collaboration and communication within social settings contribute significantly to cognitive growth. The dynamic interplay of ideas, problem-solving, and shared experiences enhances cognitive flexibility and creativity. The collective intelligence forged through social engagement becomes a catalyst for continuous intellectual development.

Immersive experiences through travel expose the mind to new environments, cultures, and ways of life. This exposure challenges preconceptions, broadening one's worldview and encouraging adaptability. The cognitive benefits derived from navigating unfamiliar territories contribute to a more resilient and open-minded cognitive framework.

Novel experiences, whether through social interactions or exploration of new environments, stimulate the mind by introducing novelty into routine patterns of thought. This encourages adaptability, broadening cognitive horizons and fostering a mindset that thrives on curiosity and exploration.

Spending time in natural environments offers profound restorative effects on the mind. The sights, sounds, and smells of nature provide a sensory stimulus that promotes relaxation, creativity, and overall well-being. Nature immersion becomes a therapeutic retreat, allowing the mind to unwind and rejuvenate, ultimately enhancing cognitive resilience.

In essence, the amalgamation of social interaction and nature exposure creates a dynamic environment that actively nurtures the mind. This holistic approach recognizes the reciprocal relationship between vibrant social connections and the rejuvenating embrace of nature, offering a comprehensive strategy for fostering cognitive vitality, adaptability, and holistic well-being.

Chapter 10

The Shadows of Doubt and Insecurity

Doubt, akin to an elusive shadow, stealthily infiltrates the intricate corridors of the mind, creating an atmosphere of uncertainty that permeates our thoughts and actions. Inseparable companions on life's journey, doubt, and insecurity collaboratively construct a challenging terrain where the beacon of self-belief often becomes obscured. This insightful exploration seeks to unravel the subtle nuances of doubt, presenting strategies that not only illuminate the shadows but also cultivate a resilient mindset capable of withstanding the insidious seeds of insecurity.

Doubt, with its nebulous nature, manifests in various forms questioning decisions, second-guessing abilities, or sowing seeds of hesitation. This exploration delves into the intricacies of doubt, dissecting its origins and manifestations. By understanding doubt at its core, individuals can navigate its complex pathways with a heightened awareness that transforms doubt from a formidable adversary into a navigable challenge.

Key Aspects of Doubt: Unraveling the Intricacies
Doubt, a subtle yet potent force, permeates the human psyche, influencing thoughts, decisions, and actions. Unraveling the

intricacies of doubt involves examining key aspects that shed light on its nature and impact. Here are essential dimensions to consider:

Doubt often originates from uncertainties, lack of information, or conflicting beliefs. Identifying the specific sources of doubt provides a foundation for understanding and addressing its manifestations. Doubt can manifest in various ways, from fleeting moments of hesitation to persistent questioning. Recognizing these expressions helps individuals pinpoint when doubt exerts its influence.

Doubt can create cognitive dissonance, a state of mental discomfort arising from conflicting beliefs or attitudes. Exploring this impact helps individuals navigate the mental tension caused by doubt. Doubt can hinder decision-making, leading to indecision or procrastination. Understanding how doubt affects choices is crucial for fostering confident decision-making.

Doubt often elicits emotions such as anxiety, fear, or frustration. Examining the emotional resonance of doubt allows individuals to address underlying feelings and manage emotional responses. Pervasive doubt can erode self-esteem and confidence. Recognizing how doubt influences self-perception is essential for cultivating a positive self-image.

Doubt may lead to avoidance or inaction as a protective mechanism. Understanding these behavioral patterns is crucial for breaking cycles of avoidance and fostering proactive approaches. Individuals grappling with doubt may seek reassurance from others. Recognizing this pattern allows for constructive communication and support within relationships.

Strategies for Resolution:
A critical examination of doubts involves evaluating evidence, challenging assumptions, and seeking additional information. This analytical approach aids in dispelling unfounded doubts. Actively cultivating self-confidence involves acknowledging achievements, focusing on strengths, and celebrating successes. This process counteracts the undermining effects of doubt. Establishing realistic expectations helps individuals navigate uncertainty by acknowledging that perfection is unattainable, and mistakes are part of growth.

Open communication with others about doubts fosters understanding and support. Sharing doubts can strengthen relationships and provide valuable perspectives. Doubt can influence collaborative efforts. Recognizing and addressing doubt within teams promotes a constructive and unified approach.
Lifelong Learning:

Viewing doubt as a gateway to curiosity encourages a lifelong learning mindset. Embracing the unknown becomes an opportunity for exploration and personal growth.

Understanding and dissecting these key aspects of doubt empowers individuals to navigate its complexities with resilience and self-awareness. By unraveling doubt's intricacies, individuals can cultivate a mindset that embraces uncertainty as a catalyst for growth and transformation.

The Shadows of Insecurity
Insecurity, often entwined with doubt, emerges as an intricate

companion, creating a nuanced psychological landscape. This section serves as a guide through the intricacies of insecurity, offering actionable strategies to nurture resilience. By acknowledging insecurities, embracing vulnerability, and fostering self-compassion, this exploration empowers individuals to dismantle barriers obstructing the flourishing of genuine self-belief.

The journey through doubt and insecurity requires the cultivation of illuminating strategies. Practical tools, including positive affirmations, goal setting, and cognitive reframing, are presented as beacons, piercing through the shadows cast by doubt. These strategies act as powerful allies, directing individuals toward a clearer understanding of their capabilities and fostering the seeds of self-belief.

Key Aspects of Insecurity:
Insecurity, a pervasive emotion, influences thoughts, behaviors, and relationships. To grasp its multifaceted nature, it's crucial to explore its key aspects. Here are essential dimensions that illuminate the intricacies of insecurity:

Insecurity often stems from past experiences of rejection, failure, or trauma. Identifying these root causes aids in understanding the origins of insecurity. External factors, such as societal expectations and comparison with others, can trigger feelings of inadequacy. Recognizing these triggers is essential for addressing insecurity at its source.

Insecurity often manifests through negative self-talk, reinforcing beliefs of incompetence or unworthiness. Recognizing and challenging these internal narratives is vital for cultivating a positive self-image. Insecurity may extend to physical appearance, leading to body image concerns. Addressing these concerns involves promoting self-acceptance and embracing diverse definitions of beauty.

Insecurity can influence relationship dynamics, leading to behaviors such as excessive reassurance-seeking or fear of abandonment. Understanding these patterns is crucial for fostering healthy connections. Insecure individuals may struggle with assertive communication, fearing rejection or judgment. Developing effective communication skills helps navigate interpersonal challenges.

Insecurity often contributes to impostor syndrome, where individuals doubt their accomplishments and fear being exposed as frauds. Recognizing and challenging these beliefs is essential for embracing achievements. Insecurity may manifest as a paralyzing fear of failure. Developing a growth mindset and reframing failure as a learning opportunity aids in overcoming this fear.

Insecurity is closely tied to anxiety and fear of inadequacy. Exploring these emotions allows individuals to address the underlying causes of insecurity and manage anxiety effectively. Insecurity often involves a fear of vulnerability and shame. Embracing vulnerability as a strength and challenging feelings of shame is essential for healing.

Strategies for Overcoming Insecurity:
Cultivating self-compassion involves treating oneself with kindness and understanding. Integrating self-compassion practices counteracts harsh self-judgment. Incorporating positive

affirmations helps reframe negative self-perceptions. Consistent affirmation practice reinforces a positive self-concept.

Insecurity often involves distorted thinking patterns. Identifying and challenging cognitive distortions contribute to a more realistic and positive mindset. Setting and achieving realistic goals boosts confidence and counters feelings of inadequacy. Celebrating small victories is integral to building self-assurance.

Insecurity may impact career progression. Developing skills, seeking mentorship, and acknowledging achievements contribute to professional growth. Overcoming insecurity enhances networking and collaboration skills, fostering meaningful professional relationships.

Understanding these key aspects of insecurity provides a comprehensive framework for individuals to navigate and overcome its challenges. By addressing insecurity at its roots and adopting proactive strategies, individuals can foster self-confidence, build fulfilling relationships, and embark on a journey of personal growth.

This exploration is not merely a guide through the shadows; it is a transformative journey toward self-discovery and empowerment. By unraveling the intricate nuances of doubt and offering pragmatic strategies to counteract insecurity, individuals are equipped to emerge from the shadows with a fortified mindset—one resilient to the seeds of insecurity and capable of embracing the radiant light of self-belief.

Chapter 11

The Echoes of Guilt and Shame

Guilt is an emotional and psychological experience characterized by feelings of remorse, self-reproach, and a sense of responsibility for a perceived wrongdoing or offense. It arises when an individual believes they have violated their moral or ethical standards, causing internal conflict and distress. Guilt often prompts individuals to acknowledge their actions, take responsibility, and seek ways to make amends or rectify the situation. It is a complex and multifaceted emotion that plays a crucial role in moral and ethical decision-making.

Guilt, stemming from a sense of wrongdoing, can become a relentless companion, clouding judgment, and hindering personal growth. This segment provides insights into navigating the complexities of guilt, offering strategies for introspection, acceptance, and atonement. By addressing guilt at its roots, individuals can begin to untangle themselves from its grip and embark on a journey toward self-forgiveness.

Guilt can manifest in various forms, such as:
Survivor Guilt: This occurs when an individual feels guilty for surviving a traumatic event while others did not. It is often

associated with feelings of unworthiness and the questioning of one's right to be alive.

Shame-Induced Guilt: This type of guilt is closely linked to feelings of shame, where individuals perceive themselves as fundamentally flawed or inadequate. Shame-induced guilt can be particularly challenging to overcome, as it goes beyond the specific actions and becomes ingrained in one's identity.

Cultural or Religious Guilt: Influenced by cultural or religious beliefs, this form of guilt arises when an individual perceives their actions as violating societal or religious norms. The moral compass is guided by external factors, and guilt serves as a mechanism for adherence to these values.

Interpersonal Guilt: This stems from actions that may have hurt or disappointed others. Interpersonal guilt involves a sense of responsibility for causing harm to someone else and often prompts individuals to seek forgiveness and repair damaged relationships.

Inaction Guilt: Sometimes, guilt arises from a perceived failure to act when action is needed. This form of guilt can be associated with missed opportunities or not living up to one's moral obligations.

Addressing guilt involves acknowledging and understanding its source, taking responsibility for one's actions, and actively working towards resolution. Seeking support from friends, family, or mental health professionals can be instrumental in navigating and overcoming the complex emotions associated with guilt.

The Echo of Shame:

Shame is a powerful and complex emotion characterized by a deep sense of unworthiness, humiliation, and a negative evaluation of oneself. Unlike guilt, which focuses on specific actions or behaviors, shame involves a pervasive feeling of inadequacy as a person. Individuals experiencing shame often believe that they are inherently flawed, defective, or unworthy of acceptance.

Shame, a profound and often paralyzing emotion, can cast a pervasive shadow on one's self-worth. This exploration guides individuals through the process of releasing the suffocating grip of shame. Strategies for embracing vulnerability, fostering self-compassion, and reframing negative self-perceptions are presented as powerful tools for dismantling the chains that shame imposes on the psyche.

Shame involves a negative perception of one's entire self. It goes beyond feeling regret for specific actions and extends to a global sense of personal failure. Shame often leads individuals to withdraw from others, as they may fear judgment or rejection. The isolation reinforces the belief that they are fundamentally different or defective.

Those experiencing shame engage in harsh self-criticism, creating a constant internal dialogue of self-blame and self-judgment. Shame can be accompanied by physical sensations such as blushing, lowered head, avoidance of eye contact, and a sense of shrinking or wanting to disappear. Cultural and societal expectations play a significant role in shaping the experience of shame. Certain cultures or communities may instill specific values that contribute to an individual's sense of shame.

Guilt and shame carry resonant echoes, reverberating through the intricate chambers of memory, carrying the weight of past actions and traumas. Unyielding and persistent, these echoes create an emotional undertow, dragging the mind into tumultuous cycles of self-blame and relentless recollection. This segment fearlessly confronts these echoes, offering profound insights into navigating the intricate complexities of guilt, releasing the suffocating grip of shame, and forging a transformative path toward healing from the lingering scars of past traumas.

Guilt and shame often act as emotional undercurrents, influencing thoughts, emotions, and behaviors. This exploration delves into the depths of these undercurrents, unraveling the intricate ways in which unresolved guilt and shame manifest. By understanding the emotional undertow, individuals gain clarity on the forces that drive cycles of self-blame and recurrent memories, laying the foundation for transformative change.

Overcoming shame involves self-compassion, challenging negative self-perceptions, and fostering a sense of self-worth. Therapy, support groups, and open communication with trusted individuals can be valuable resources in addressing and healing from shame.

The Effect of Reverberating Trauma
In the case of trauma, the episode of past trauma can indeed constitute a significant battle in the mind. Traumatic experiences can leave a lasting impact on an individual's mental and emotional well-being, creating internal struggles that may persist over time. The effects of trauma can manifest in various ways, influencing thoughts, emotions, and behaviors.

Individuals may experience intrusive memories, flashbacks, or nightmares related to the traumatic event. These recurring thoughts can disrupt daily life and contribute to heightened stress and anxiety. Trauma can intrude into cognitive processes, impacting concentration, memory, and decision-making. Individuals may struggle with a constant replay of the traumatic event in their minds.

Trauma often leads to intense emotional distress, including feelings of fear, anger, sadness, or numbness. Managing these emotions becomes a constant internal challenge. To cope with the pain and distress associated with trauma, individuals may develop avoidance behaviors. This can include avoiding certain places, people, or activities that trigger memories of the trauma.

Past trauma can contribute to a negative self-perception, with individuals blaming themselves for the event or feeling a pervasive sense of guilt and shame. The effects of trauma can extend to interpersonal relationships, making it challenging to trust others, form connections, or maintain healthy boundaries.

Addressing the battle in the mind caused by past trauma often involves therapeutic interventions, such as trauma-focused therapy, counseling, and support groups. Recognizing the impact of trauma and seeking professional help are crucial steps toward healing and reclaiming mental well-being.

Trauma, woven into the echoes of memory, requires a delicate and intentional approach toward healing. This segment acknowledges the impact of past traumas and introduces pathways for healing, including therapy, mindfulness practices, and self-care. By addressing trauma with empathy and courage, individuals can initiate a transformative journey towards reclaiming agency over their narratives.

Confronting echoes is not an easy task, but it is a courageous step towards reclaiming one's mental landscape. By navigating the complexities of guilt, releasing the grip of shame, and forging a path toward healing from past traumas, individuals can find the strength to rewrite their narratives and embark on a journey toward emotional liberation and resilience.

Chapter 12

The Spectrum of Anxiety and Paranoia

Anxiety is a natural and adaptive response that serves as a vital part of the human experience. It encompasses a range of emotional and physiological reactions triggered by perceived threats or challenges. This complex and nuanced phenomenon can manifest in various forms, from everyday worries to more intense feelings of fear and apprehension.

At its milder end, anxiety involves common stressors related to work, relationships, or daily responsibilities—everyday worries that are a normal part of life. As anxiety intensifies, individuals may experience generalized anxiety, characterized by excessive worry and tension about various aspects of life. This state can become persistent and challenging to control, impacting overall well-being.

Moving along the spectrum, anxiety can escalate to phobias or panic attacks. Specific fears or situations may trigger intense anxiety, leading to physical symptoms such as a rapid heartbeat, shortness of breath, and a sense of impending doom. Social anxiety is another subset, where individuals fear judgment or scrutiny in social interactions, impacting relationships and social engagement.

In some cases, anxiety may manifest as obsessive-compulsive traits, involving repetitive behaviors or rituals aimed at alleviating distress. In the end, paranoia arises, characterized by persistent and irrational beliefs that others are plotting against or spying on the individual. This condition can cause considerable distress and disrupt daily functioning.

What is Paranoia?
Paranoia is a mental state characterized by persistent and irrational suspicions and fears that individuals are the target of conspiracies or malevolent actions by others. Paranoia often leads to heightened vigilance, distrust, and an overwhelming sense of being threatened.

Individuals experiencing paranoia may interpret innocent actions or events as deliberate threats against them, even when there is no evidence to support such beliefs. This state of heightened suspicion can significantly impact daily life, leading to social withdrawal, strained relationships, and impaired overall functioning.

Paranoia exists on the more end of the anxiety spectrum and often requires careful evaluation and support from mental health professionals to address the underlying concerns and help individuals manage their distress.

The spectrum of anxiety and paranoia encompasses a range of emotional experiences and cognitive states that can significantly impact an individual's mental well-being. Anxiety and paranoia, while distinct, share common threads in navigating the intricate landscape of the mind.

Key aspects of the spectrum of anxiety and paranoia:
Every day we often find ourselves contending with commonplace concerns and stresses that are part and parcel of daily life. These worries may revolve around various aspects such as work-related pressures, interpersonal relationships, or the demands and responsibilities inherent in day-to-day living.

The range of anxiety and paranoia comprises the variety of everyday stressors that people face, including the wide range of obstacles that may cause them to feel anxious or tense as they go through the complexities of their everyday lives. Everyday concerns, such as making job deadlines and preserving happy relationships, provide a common background to the human experience, gently affecting mental states and adding to the larger fabric of worry.

Also, we may find ourselves grappling with the complexities of generalized anxiety, marked by an overall sense of excessive worry and tension that extends across various facets of life. This state of heightened anxiety is not limited to specific triggers or stressors but manifests as a pervasive, persistent apprehension about a range of circumstances and outcomes. Unlike everyday worries, generalized anxiety involves a more profound and enduring sense of unease, often proving challenging to control or mitigate.

The inclination for people to predict bad things to happen, no matter how likely they are, is a defining feature of generalized anxiety. This ongoing anxiety can have a substantial negative effect on day-to-day functioning, decision-making, and vulnerability perception. The mind, under the grip of generalized anxiety, may constantly generate scenarios of potential threats or dangers, leading to a continuous cycle of worry.

Progressing along the spectrum, anxiety can escalate to more intense manifestations, including the development of phobias and the occurrence of panic attacks. In this segment, individuals may experience heightened anxiety specifically tied to certain fears or situations, resulting in an overwhelming and often debilitating response.

Phobias are characterized by an intense and irrational fear of specific objects, activities, or situations. These fears can vary widely, encompassing anything from common phobias like fear of heights (acrophobia) or fear of spiders (arachnophobia) to more specific phobias related to particular situations or stimuli. When confronted with the phobic trigger, individuals may experience heightened anxiety, accompanied by physical symptoms such as a rapid heartbeat, shortness of breath, trembling, and a compelling urge to escape the situation.

Panic attacks, on the other hand, represent acute episodes of intense fear or discomfort that can arise suddenly and unpredictably. These episodes are characterized by a surge of overwhelming anxiety accompanied by a range of physical symptoms. Individuals undergoing a panic attack may experience chest pain, dizziness, sweating, and a sense of impending doom. The intensity of these symptoms can be so severe that individuals may feel as though they are losing control or experiencing a life-threatening situation.

Within the spectrum of anxiety, a distinctive subset is social anxiety, a condition marked by an intense fear of social situations.

Individuals grappling with social anxiety experience an overwhelming concern about being negatively judged, embarrassed, or scrutinized during interactions with others. This heightened fear can extend to a variety of social settings, including parties, gatherings, and even routine encounters.

Social anxiety can significantly impact relationships and limit one's ability to engage socially. The fear of perceived judgment or negative evaluation often leads individuals to avoid social situations altogether, creating a pattern of isolation and hindering the development of meaningful connections. Everyday activities, such as speaking in public, attending social events, or even making small talk, may evoke distressing levels of anxiety for those affected by social anxiety.

Moving along the spectrum of anxiety, another facet involves obsessive-compulsive traits, a condition characterized by repetitive behaviors or rituals undertaken to alleviate persistent anxiety. Individuals grappling with obsessive-compulsive traits often find themselves trapped in a cycle of compulsive actions driven by intrusive, distressing thoughts.

These compulsive behaviors can take various forms, such as repeated handwashing, checking, counting, or arranging objects in specific patterns. While engaging in these rituals may offer temporary relief from anxiety, it becomes a double-edged sword as the need for repetition can intensify over time. The cycle of obsession and compulsion can significantly interfere with daily functioning and impact the overall quality of life. .

Advancing towards the more end of the anxiety spectrum, paranoia manifests as persistent and irrational beliefs that others are conspiring against or surveilling the individual. In this state, heightened suspicion and mistrust become defining features, creating a pervasive sense of threat and danger in various aspects of life.

Individuals experiencing paranoia may harbor unfounded beliefs that they are being watched, followed, or targeted, even in the absence of credible evidence. These intrusive thoughts can lead to significant distress, anxiety, and a heightened state of vigilance. The impact on daily functioning can be profound, as individuals may alter their behavior, routines, or social interactions in an attempt to mitigate perceived threats.

Navigating the spectrum of anxiety and paranoia is a multifaceted process that involves comprehensive understanding, identification of triggers, and the development of effective coping mechanisms. Here are ways to overcome anxiety and paranoia:

Understanding the Roots: Anxiety often stems from a combination of genetic, environmental, and neurological factors. It can be triggered by stressors, trauma, or imbalances in brain chemistry. Paranoia may have origins in past traumas, abusive experiences, or deep-seated insecurities. It can also be associated with mental health conditions such as paranoid personality disorder or schizophrenia.

Identifying Triggers: Everyday worries, work-related stress, relationship issues, and financial concerns can trigger anxiety. Identifying specific stressors is crucial for targeted intervention. Paranoia triggers may include social interactions, perceived threats, or situations reminiscent of past traumas. Understanding these triggers helps in developing tailored coping strategies.

Developing Coping Mechanisms: Mindfulness and Relaxation Techniques: Practices like deep breathing, meditation, and progressive muscle relaxation can calm the mind and reduce anxiety. Identifying and challenging negative thought patterns can reshape cognitive responses to stressors.

Other management techniques include Regular exercise, proper sleep, and a healthy lifestyle contribute to overall stress reduction.

Paranoia Coping Mechanisms: Encouraging individuals to objectively evaluate their thoughts and question whether the perceived threat is real can help challenge paranoid beliefs. Psychotherapy, particularly cognitive-behavioral therapy (CBT), can address distorted thinking patterns associated with paranoia. Establishing a supportive network can provide a reality check and emotional reassurance. Therapy and Counseling: Mental health professionals, such as psychologists or counselors, can guide individuals in exploring the root causes of anxiety and paranoia and developing coping strategies.

Combining various strategies, including therapy, lifestyle changes, and prescribed medication, if necessary, offers a holistic approach to managing anxiety and paranoia. Encouraging individuals to actively participate in their mental health journey empowers them to develop a personalized toolkit for navigating the spectrum of these challenging emotions.

In summary, navigating the spectrum of anxiety and paranoia involves a personalized and holistic approach, encompassing understanding, identification, coping mechanisms, and professional support.

Chapter 13

The Shadows of Depression

Depression is a complex and pervasive mental health condition characterized by persistent feelings of sadness, hopelessness, and a lack of interest or pleasure in activities. It goes beyond the normal fluctuations in mood that people experience and can significantly impact various aspects of daily life, including work, relationships, and physical health.

There are several types of depression, each with its unique characteristics and symptoms. Some of the common types of depression are:

Major Depressive Disorder (MDD):
Major Depressive Disorder, or clinical depression, is the most common type. It involves persistent feelings of sadness, hopelessness, and a lack of interest in activities. Symptoms include changes in sleep patterns, appetite, and energy levels, as well as feelings of worthlessness and difficulty concentrating. Treatment may involve therapy, medication, or a combination of both.

Persistent Depressive Disorder (Dysthymia):

Persistent Depressive Disorder is characterized by a long-term, chronic form of depression. The symptoms are less severe than MDD but last for a more extended period. Chronic feelings of sadness, low energy, and a lack of interest or pleasure in activities. Treatment often includes therapy, and medication may be prescribed in some cases.

Bipolar Disorder (Manic-Depressive Illness):
Bipolar Disorder involves alternating periods of depression and mania or hypomania (a less severe form of mania). Depressive episodes are similar to MDD, while manic episodes involve elevated mood, increased energy, and impulsive behavior. Mood stabilizers, medication, and therapy are common treatments.

Seasonal Affective Disorder (SAD):
SAD is a type of depression that occurs seasonally, typically in the fall and winter when there is less sunlight. Symptoms include low energy, irritability, changes in sleep and appetite, and a persistent feeling of sadness. Light therapy, psychotherapy, and medication may be recommended.

Psychotic Depression:
Psychotic Depression combines severe depressive symptoms with psychotic features, such as hallucinations or delusions. Individuals may experience breaks from reality, including false beliefs or sensory experiences. Medication and psychotherapy are often used, and hospitalization may be necessary in severe cases.

Postpartum Depression:
Postpartum Depression occurs after giving birth and involves feelings of extreme sadness, anxiety, and exhaustion. Symptoms

may include mood swings, changes in sleep and appetite, and difficulty bonding with the newborn. Therapy, support groups, and, in some cases, medication are recommended.

Premenstrual Dysphoric Disorder (PMDD):
PMDD is a severe form of premenstrual syndrome (PMS) characterized by intense mood swings, irritability, and depression. Emotional and physical symptoms typically occur in the week or two before menstruation. Medication, lifestyle changes, and therapy may be used to manage symptoms.

Depression is a complex and varied condition, and individuals may experience a combination of symptoms from different types of depression. Diagnosis and treatment should be tailored to each individual's specific needs and circumstances. Seeking professional help is crucial for accurate diagnosis and effective management.

Key aspects of depression include:
Individuals with depression often experience a deep and prolonged sense of sadness or emptiness. This emotional state may persist for weeks, months, or even longer. A notable feature of depression is the diminished interest or pleasure in once enjoyable activities. Hobbies, social interactions, and even routine tasks may no longer bring the same satisfaction.

Depression can affect sleep, leading to either insomnia or excessive sleeping. Disruptions in the sleep-wake cycle contribute to the overall sense of fatigue and lethargy. Significant changes in appetite and weight are common symptoms of depression. Some individuals may experience a loss of appetite and weight loss, while others may find comfort in overeating, leading to weight gain.

Individuals with depression often report persistent feelings of fatigue and a general lack of energy. Even simple tasks may feel overwhelming. Depression can impact cognitive functions, making it challenging to concentrate, make decisions, or remember things.

Individuals with depression may harbor intense feelings of worthlessness, guilt, or self-blame. These negative thoughts contribute to the overall burden of the condition. Depression can manifest in physical symptoms such as headaches, stomach aches, and other unexplained aches and pains.

Episodes of depression:
Episodes of depressive states refer to distinct periods during which individuals experience the pervasive and debilitating symptoms associated with depression. These episodes are characterized by a profound and persistent low mood, along with a range of emotional, cognitive, and physical manifestations. Each episode can vary in intensity, duration, and specific symptoms, but they collectively contribute to the overall impact of depression on an individual's well-being.

Key Features of Episodes of Depressive States:
Profound Sadness: Profound sadness is characterized by an intense emotional state that surpasses the typical fluctuations in mood experienced in everyday life. In this context, individuals undergoing profound sadness encounter an overwhelming and pervasive feeling of sorrow, grief, or unhappiness that goes beyond the usual ups and downs of emotions.

This emotional experience is often all-encompassing, affecting various aspects of an individual's life, including their thoughts, behaviors, and overall well-being. It can manifest as a heavy, burdensome feeling that lingers and colors one's perception of the world. Unlike ordinary moments of feeling down, profound sadness tends to be more persistent, enduring for more extended periods, and significantly impacting a person's ability to find joy or satisfaction in daily activities.

Recognizing profound sadness is crucial, as it can be indicative of underlying emotional struggles, mental health challenges, or specific life circumstances that require attention and support. Addressing this profound sadness may involve seeking professional help, engaging in therapeutic interventions, and exploring healthy coping mechanisms to navigate and overcome the emotional weight it brings.

Loss of Interest and Pleasure: Loss of interest and pleasure, often referred to as anhedonia, is a prominent feature of depressive episodes. Anhedonia manifests as a pervasive and profound inability to derive joy, satisfaction, or interest from activities that were previously enjoyable or fulfilling. It goes beyond the ordinary fluctuations in mood and represents a significant shift in one's ability to experience pleasure.

Individuals experiencing anhedonia may find that hobbies, social interactions, and other activities that once brought them happiness or a sense of accomplishment no longer evoke the same positive emotions. The loss of interest can extend to various aspects of life, affecting both personal and social spheres. This diminished capacity to experience pleasure can contribute to a sense of emptiness, detachment, and overall dissatisfaction with life.

Recognizing anhedonia is crucial in understanding the impact of depressive states, as it is a key diagnostic criterion for depressive disorders. Addressing this loss of interest and pleasure often involves therapeutic interventions, lifestyle adjustments, and support from mental health professionals. Identifying and treating anhedonia is integral to restoring a person's ability to engage in meaningful and enjoyable activities, promoting overall well-being.

Fatigue and Low Energy: Fatigue and low energy are pervasive symptoms associated with depressive states. Individuals grappling with depression often experience an overwhelming sense of tiredness, lethargy, and a notable decline in both physical and mental energy levels. These symptoms go beyond the ordinary tiredness that can result from a lack of sleep or strenuous physical activity.

The fatigue associated with depression can manifest as a persistent feeling of exhaustion, making even simple tasks seem daunting. Individuals may find themselves struggling to muster the energy needed to engage in daily activities, work, or social interactions. This fatigue can contribute to a sense of inertia, further amplifying the challenges associated with depression.

The interplay between mental and physical energy is crucial in understanding the holistic impact of depression. Low energy levels can hinder concentration, impair decision-making, and diminish overall motivation. Consequently, individuals may withdraw from activities, isolate themselves, and face difficulties in maintaining a routine.

Recognizing the presence of fatigue and low energy is vital for both self-awareness and effective mental health management. Treatment approaches for depression often include interventions to address these symptoms, encompassing a combination of therapy, lifestyle adjustments, and, in some cases, medication. By addressing fatigue, individuals can take crucial steps toward restoring their overall vitality and well-being.

Sleep Disturbances: Sleep disturbances are common and impactful features of depressive states, manifesting as either insomnia or excessive sleep. These disruptions often lead to significant alterations in normal sleep patterns, exacerbating the challenges associated with depression.

Insomnia, characterized by difficulty falling asleep, staying asleep, or experiencing non-restorative sleep, is a prevalent symptom in depressive episodes. Individuals may find themselves lying awake at night, their minds racing with negative thoughts, worries, or feelings of hopelessness. The persistent struggle to initiate or maintain sleep can contribute to increased fatigue, irritability, and heightened emotional distress.

Conversely, some individuals may experience hypersomnia, marked by prolonged sleep durations or excessive daytime sleepiness. The desire to escape the challenges of wakefulness may lead individuals to spend extended hours in bed, yet the quality of sleep remains compromised. Excessive sleep can contribute to a cycle of disengagement from daily activities, social interactions, and responsibilities.

These disruptions in sleep patterns further underscore the intricate interplay between mental health and the circadian rhythms that regulate sleep-wake cycles. The bidirectional relationship between depression and sleep disturbances highlights the importance of addressing both aspects for comprehensive mental health care.

Effective management of sleep disturbances often involves a multi-faceted approach. Therapeutic interventions, such as cognitive-behavioral therapy for insomnia (CBT-I), may be employed to address maladaptive sleep patterns. Additionally, lifestyle adjustments, sleep hygiene practices, and, in some cases, medications may be recommended to restore healthier sleep patterns and contribute to overall well-being in individuals experiencing depressive episodes.

Changes in Appetite: Depressive states frequently manifest in notable changes in appetite, contributing to variations in weight. Individuals experiencing these fluctuations may either exhibit a significant decrease in appetite, resulting in noticeable weight loss or conversely, an increase in appetite leading to weight gain. These alterations in eating patterns represent key features of depressive episodes.

Individuals grappling with depressive states may find themselves experiencing a notable loss of appetite. The pleasure and interest in food may diminish, leading to reduced meal consumption. This diminished desire for nourishment, coupled with the emotional and physical toll of depression, can contribute to weight loss over time.

The lack of interest in eating often parallels other symptoms of depression, such as fatigue, lethargy, and a sense of hopelessness.

Increased Appetite and Weight Gain: On the contrary, some individuals may encounter heightened appetite during depressive episodes, leading to increased food intake. This form of emotional eating can serve as a coping mechanism, providing temporary relief from the emotional distress associated with depression. The types of foods chosen during such episodes may lean towards comfort or high-calorie options. Consequently, this increase in caloric intake can result in weight gain.

These changes in appetite are not only indicative of the physical toll depression takes on the body but also underscore the intricate relationship between mood and eating behaviors. The bidirectional influence between emotional well-being and dietary habits necessitates a comprehensive approach to address both mental health and nutritional aspects. Collaborative efforts involving mental health professionals, nutritionists, and healthcare providers may be instrumental in developing tailored strategies to manage these fluctuations in appetite and support individuals in their journey toward mental and physical well-being.

Feelings of Worthlessness or Guilt: During depressive states, individuals often grapple with profound and irrational feelings of worthlessness, guilt, or self-blame. These emotional burdens extend beyond normal fluctuations in mood, creating a pervasive and distressing internal dialogue that erodes self-esteem.

Depressive episodes can plunge individuals into a deep sense of worthlessness, where they perceive themselves as inherently flawed or devoid of value. These feelings are affecting how people perceive their personal abilities, achievements, and overall self-worth. The mind becomes entangled in a distorted narrative that reinforces a negative self-image, making it challenging for individuals to recognize their inherent values and strengths.

Depression often magnifies perceived personal shortcomings, leading to intense guilt and self-blame. Individuals may irrationally assign responsibility to themselves for circumstances beyond their control or attribute exaggerated fault to their actions. This self-flagellation contributes to a cycle of negative thoughts and emotions, reinforcing the sense of unworthiness. The weight of guilt becomes a heavy burden, hindering the ability to navigate daily life and engage in activities that once brought joy.

Addressing these profound feelings of worthlessness and guilt within the context of depression requires a multifaceted approach. Mental health interventions, such as psychotherapy, can provide a safe space for individuals to explore and challenge distorted beliefs about themselves. Additionally, building a support system that includes friends, family, and mental health professionals is crucial in helping individuals reframe their self-perceptions and embark on a path toward healing and self-compassion.

Difficulty Concentrating: Amid depressive episodes, individuals frequently grapple with the notable challenge of concentrating and maintaining cognitive focus. This cognitive impairment extends beyond momentary distractions or lapses in attention; it becomes a pervasive obstacle that interferes with daily functioning.

Depression casts a shadow over the ability to concentrate, diminishing the capacity to direct attention and engage in tasks. Individuals may find it arduous to focus on work, studies, or even simple daily activities. The mind becomes clouded by a persistent fog, making it difficult to sift through information, process thoughts, and complete tasks efficiently. This diminished concentration can have cascading effects on various aspects of life, affecting productivity and exacerbating feelings of frustration and inadequacy.

The cognitive impact of depressive states extends to decision-making processes. Individuals may experience indecision, hesitation, or a general sense of being overwhelmed when faced with choices. Even seemingly straightforward decisions can become sources of stress and mental fatigue. This can lead to avoidance of decision-making altogether, further hindering progress in personal and professional spheres.

Depressive episodes often bring about memory challenges, disrupting the normal processes of encoding, storing, and retrieving information. Forgetfulness and difficulty recalling details of recent events or conversations are common manifestations. This memory impairment can lead to feelings of frustration and contribute to a sense of cognitive decline.

Navigating the difficulty of concentrating during depressive episodes necessitates a comprehensive approach. Seeking professional guidance through therapy or counseling can help individuals develop strategies to improve focus and manage cognitive challenges. Incorporating mindfulness practices, such as meditation, may also contribute to enhancing cognitive clarity and concentration. Additionally, creating a structured routine and breaking tasks into manageable steps can aid in mitigating the impact of cognitive impairment associated with depression.

Physical Symptoms: Within the realm of depressive episodes, the impact extends beyond emotional and cognitive realms to manifest as tangible physical symptoms, contributing to the overall complexity of the experience.

A common physical manifestation of depression is headaches. Individuals may experience persistent or recurrent headaches, often characterized by tension or pressure. These headaches can contribute to a sense of physical discomfort, adding a layer to the overall burden of depressive states.

Depression can intertwine with the digestive system, giving rise to various issues. Some individuals may encounter changes in appetite, leading to digestive discomfort or irregularities. This can manifest as stomach aches, nausea, or disruptions in bowel habits. The intricate connection between the mind and the gut becomes apparent as emotional struggles manifest physically.

A pervasive sense of bodily discomfort is another facet of the physical toll that depression can take. Individuals may describe feeling achy, tense, or generally unwell. This discomfort is not localized but permeates throughout the body, contributing to an overall sense of malaise.

Understanding and addressing these physical symptoms is crucial in comprehensive depression management. Seeking medical advice can help rule out underlying medical conditions contributing to these symptoms. Engaging in regular physical activity, even in small increments, can positively impact both physical and mental well-being. Additionally, adopting stress-reduction techniques, such as deep breathing or progressive muscle relaxation, may alleviate physical discomfort associated with depressive episodes.

Social Withdrawal: One of the hallmark manifestations of depression is the withdrawal from once-enjoyed social activities. Hobbies, gatherings, and events that once brought joy may lose their allure. Individuals in depressive states often find it challenging to engage in social interactions, contributing to a sense of detachment from the vibrant nature of social life.

The inclination toward isolation is a common feature of depressive episodes. Individuals may prefer solitude, retreating into the comfort of their own space. Isolation can intensify feelings of loneliness and exacerbate the sense of being disconnected from the support and understanding of others.

The emotional weight of depression can create a perceptual barrier, leading to a profound sense of disconnection from others. Even in the presence of loved ones, individuals may feel emotionally distant, as if a metaphorical chasm separates them from the understanding and empathy of those around them.

Addressing social withdrawal in depression requires a nuanced approach. Encouraging gentle and understanding communication is essential. Loved ones can play a crucial role by offering support without judgment and providing a reassuring presence. Gradual reintegration into social activities, even in small steps, can contribute to breaking the cycle of isolation. Professional intervention, such as therapy or counseling, may also provide valuable guidance in navigating the complexities of social withdrawal associated with depressive states.

Suicidal Thoughts: In the shadows of profound despair, the haunting specter of suicidal thoughts emerges as a deeply distressing aspect of mental health struggles. Suicidal ideation often involves persistent thoughts of self-harm or inflicting physical pain. Individuals may grapple with a profound sense of hopelessness, viewing self-harm as a means to cope with overwhelming emotional pain.

In more severe cases, individuals may contemplate suicide as a way to escape the relentless anguish that characterizes their mental state. These thoughts can evolve into detailed plans, intensifying the urgency for immediate intervention and support. Suicidal thoughts can be a desperate cry for help, signaling an individual's inability to navigate the overwhelming darkness within. It's crucial to recognize these thoughts as a call for support and intervention, urging loved ones and professionals to provide timely assistance.

Addressing suicidal thoughts requires swift and compassionate action. If you or someone you know is experiencing these thoughts, seek professional help immediately. Mental health hotlines, crisis intervention services, and emergency medical services can provide vital support. Engaging in open and non-judgmental conversations, encouraging professional intervention, and creating a supportive environment are essential steps in fostering hope and recovery. Remember, there is help available, and reaching out is a courageous step towards healing.

Depressive episodes can vary in duration, lasting from a few weeks to several months. Some individuals may experience recurrent episodes throughout their lives, while others may have isolated occurrences. The frequency and severity of these episodes contribute to the overall diagnosis and management of depressive disorders.

Effective treatment for episodes of depressive states often involves a combination of psychotherapy, medication, lifestyle changes, and support from mental health professionals. Recognizing the symptoms, seeking timely intervention, and establishing a comprehensive treatment plan are crucial steps in managing depressive episodes and promoting mental well-being.

It's important to note that depression varies in severity, and its causes are multifaceted, involving genetic, biological, environmental, and psychological factors. Seeking professional help, such as therapy or medication, is crucial for effectively managing and treating depression.

THE METAMORPHOSIS OF THE MIND

Chapter 14

The Abyss of Suicidal Thoughts

Suicidal thoughts, also known as suicidal ideation, refer to the contemplation or preoccupation with thoughts of ending one's own life. These thoughts can vary in intensity, duration, and frequency, ranging from fleeting considerations to persistent and intrusive ideation. Suicidal thoughts are a serious and concerning aspect of mental health, indicating significant emotional distress and psychological pain. It's crucial for individuals experiencing such thoughts to seek professional help, as timely intervention, support, and appropriate mental health care are essential for their well-being and safety.

Suicidal thoughts can have various triggers and origins, and they may develop over time due to a combination of factors. Some common contributors include:

Mental Health Conditions, comprising disorders such as depression, anxiety, bipolar disorder, and other mood disorders, represent a critical factor amplifying the vulnerability to suicidal thoughts. These conditions, often characterized by profound disturbances in emotional well-being, cognitive functioning, and behavioral patterns, create a heightened risk for individuals to experience thoughts of self-harm or suicide.

Depression, a pervasive and debilitating mental health condition, can cast a shadow over one's perception of life, robbing individuals of the ability to find joy or meaning in their existence. The overwhelming sense of hopelessness and despair that accompanies depression can increase the risk of contemplating suicide as a way to escape relentless emotional pain.

Anxiety disorders, marked by excessive worry, fear, and nervousness, can contribute to a sense of entrapment and desperation. The relentless nature of anxiety, if left unmanaged, may exacerbate feelings of helplessness, ultimately elevating the risk of suicidal ideation.

Bipolar disorder, characterized by extreme mood swings between depressive and manic states, introduces unique challenges. In the depressive phase, individuals may grapple with intense sadness and hopelessness, mirroring the experiences of those with major depressive disorder. Conversely, during manic episodes, impulsive and risky behaviors may escalate the danger associated with suicidal thoughts.

These mental health conditions intertwine with the fabric of an individual's psyche, creating a complex landscape where emotions, thoughts, and behaviors become intertwined. The exploration of suicidal thoughts in the context of mental health conditions emphasizes the crucial need for timely and comprehensive mental health interventions. Addressing the root causes of these conditions through therapeutic approaches, medication, and support networks becomes imperative in mitigating the risk and guiding individuals toward a path of healing and resilience.

Trauma, whether stemming from past experiences, abuse, or significant life events, constitutes a potent precursor to the emergence of suicidal thoughts. Individuals who have endured traumatic incidents may find themselves grappling with the enduring impact of these experiences, creating a profound sense of emotional distress and vulnerability.

Past traumatic experiences, ranging from physical or emotional abuse to accidents or witnessing distressing events, can leave deep scars on the psyche. The lingering effects of trauma may manifest in the form of post-traumatic stress disorder (PTSD) or other trauma-related conditions, intensifying the risk of suicidal thoughts. The intrusive memories, flashbacks, and emotional upheaval associated with trauma can overwhelm individuals, prompting them to seek an escape from their painful reality.

Moreover, a history of significant life events such as loss, bereavement, financial setbacks, or relationship breakdowns can act as catalysts for suicidal ideation. The profound disruptions caused by these events can trigger overwhelming feelings of despair, hopelessness, and a perceived inability to cope with life's challenges.

Understanding the intricate link between trauma and suicidal thoughts underscores the importance of trauma-informed care and mental health support. Therapeutic interventions that address the impact of trauma, coupled with a compassionate and empathetic approach, play a pivotal role in helping individuals navigate the complex aftermath of traumatic experiences and work towards healing and resilience.

Substance Abuse, encompassing the misuse of alcohol or drugs, intertwines with the intricate nature of mental health, intensifying the risk of suicidal ideation. Substance abuse serves as a complex contributor to the development and exacerbation of existing mental health issues, creating a precarious intersection where vulnerability and distress converge.

Alcohol and drug misuse can act as a double-edged sword, offering temporary relief from emotional pain while simultaneously exacerbating mental health challenges. The impact of substances on cognitive function and emotional regulation can distort an individual's perception of reality, intensifying feelings of despair and hopelessness.

Moreover, substance abuse can alter brain chemistry, amplifying the effects of mental health conditions such as depression or anxiety. The intoxicating allure of substances may serve as a coping mechanism for individuals grappling with emotional turmoil, providing a temporary escape from their internal struggles.

Recognizing the intricate link between substance abuse and suicidal ideation underscores the importance of integrated treatment approaches. Comprehensive interventions addressing both mental health and substance misuse, such as dual-diagnosis treatment programs, play a crucial role in untangling the complex interplay between these factors. Supportive therapy, counseling, and substance abuse rehabilitation can empower individuals to navigate the challenging terrain of dual challenges, fostering a pathway toward recovery and renewed mental well-being.

Chronic Pain or Illness manifests as a silent antagonist, weaving threads of persistent physical distress that intertwine with the fabric of mental well-being. The burden of enduring physical health challenges or grappling with chronic pain can cast a looming shadow on an individual's psyche, potentially paving the way for the emergence of suicidal thoughts.

The relentless nature of chronic conditions creates a profound impact on various facets of life, from daily functioning to overall quality of life. Coping with the persistent demands of managing a chronic illness or navigating the throes of chronic pain can erode an individual's resilience, amplifying feelings of despair and hopelessness.

The intricate relationship between chronic pain, illness, and suicidal ideation underscores the need for holistic and compassionate healthcare approaches. Addressing both the physical and mental dimensions of health becomes imperative, with a focus on pain management, symptom relief, and psychological support.

In such cases, healthcare professionals play a pivotal role in collaboratively developing tailored interventions that acknowledge the interconnectedness of physical and mental well-being. Integrative strategies encompassing pain management techniques, mental health support, and fostering a sense of empowerment over one's health journey can serve as crucial components in alleviating the burden of chronic pain or illness and mitigating the risk of suicidal thoughts.

Feelings of Isolation unfold as a poignant chapter in the narrative of mental health struggles, where the absence of social connection casts a profound impact on one's emotional landscape. The intricate interplay between solitude and despair creates a breeding ground for feelings of hopelessness, potentially steering an individual toward the tumultuous waters of suicidal thoughts.

The human psyche inherently craves social bonds, and when these bonds are strained or severed, the repercussions reverberate through one's emotional resilience. The absence of a supportive social network can amplify feelings of despair, alienation, and a profound sense of being unmoored.

Navigating the complexities of isolation-induced despair requires a multi-faceted approach. Interventions that foster social connection, whether through community engagement, support groups, or rebuilding interpersonal relationships, become instrumental in breaking the chains of isolation. Cultivating a sense of belonging and purpose, even in seemingly small interactions, contributes significantly to mitigating the risk of suicidal thoughts.

Addressing feelings of isolation mandates a collective effort from individuals, communities, and mental health professionals alike. By recognizing the pivotal role of social connectedness in mental well-being, society can weave a safety net that catches those at risk, offering solace, understanding, and a pathway toward healing.

Loss or Grief unfolds as a poignant chapter in the human experience, where the weight of significant losses becomes a formidable trigger for the emergence of suicidal thoughts. The journey through grief, marked by the death of a loved one or the shattering of significant relationships, navigates delicate terrain that can lead individuals to the precipice of despair.

Grief, a universal response to loss, encapsulates a spectrum of emotions, from profound sadness to anger, confusion, and a sense of emptiness. In the wake of loss, individuals grapple not only with the tangible absence of what once was but also with the void left in the fabric of their emotional world. The process of mourning, while natural, can spiral into the depths of despair, especially when compounded by the complexities of personal struggles and mental health challenges.

Navigating the entanglement of grief-induced vulnerability necessitates a compassionate and nuanced approach. Support systems, including friends, family, and mental health professionals, play a pivotal role in offering solace and understanding during these tumultuous times. Acknowledging the depth of pain and creating spaces for expression becomes crucial in preventing the evolution of grief into entrenched despair and suicidal thoughts.

Recognizing the intertwined nature of grief and mental health, society can foster environments that prioritize empathy, active listening, and open conversations about loss. By weaving a supportive network, individuals traversing the landscape of grief can find strength, resilience, and the collective embrace needed to weather the storm of emotions and navigate toward healing.

Financial Strain: This segment of the exploration illuminates the intricate relationship between economic hardships and the emergence of suicidal thoughts. When individuals find themselves ensnared in the clutches of severe financial difficulties, a disheartening cycle of desperation and hopelessness can unfold, casting a dark shadow on their mental well-being.

The impact of financial strain on mental health is profound, as economic challenges permeate various aspects of life. Individuals grappling with the weight of financial burdens may experience heightened stress, anxiety, and a pervasive sense of uncertainty about the future. The relentless pressure to meet financial obligations, coupled with the potential erosion of personal and social support structures, can create an environment conducive to the development of suicidal thoughts.

Understanding the interconnected nature of financial strain and mental health underscores the importance of comprehensive support systems. Initiatives aimed at providing financial literacy, employment opportunities, and mental health resources can contribute to alleviating the burdens that individuals face. Furthermore, fostering a culture that destigmatizes discussions around financial challenges and mental health encourages open dialogue and reduces the isolation often associated with economic difficulties.

By addressing the multifaceted dimensions of financial strain and its impact on mental well-being, society can strive to create a more empathetic and supportive environment. Such efforts play a crucial role in breaking the chains of despair that often accompany severe economic hardships, offering pathways to resilience, recovery, and liberation from the throes of suicidal thoughts.

Genetic Factors: A family history steeped in mental health issues or suicide serves as a complex backdrop, intertwining genetic predispositions with environmental influences to create a potentially heightened risk.

Heritability refers to the proportion of variation in a trait (such as suicidal thoughts) that can be attributed to genetic factors. Studies involving family history, twin, and adoption data suggest that suicidal thoughts and behaviors have a genetic component. Heritability estimates for suicidal thoughts range from 30% to 55%.

Researchers have identified specific candidate genes associated with suicidal tendencies. These genes are involved in neurotransmitter regulation, stress response, and neural plasticity. Examples include variations in the serotonin transporter gene (SLC6A4) and the brain-derived neurotrophic factor gene (BDNF).

Epigenetic modifications (changes in gene expression without altering the DNA sequence) also play a role. Stress, trauma, and adverse life events can lead to epigenetic changes that influence susceptibility to suicidal thoughts.

Genetic predisposition interacts with environmental factors (such as childhood adversity, substance abuse, or social isolation). The combination of genetic vulnerability and environmental stressors contributes to the risk of suicidal ideation.

Suicidal thoughts arise from a complex interplay of genetic, psychological, social, and environmental factors. Genetic predisposition alone does not determine suicidal tendencies; it interacts with other influences.

Researchers have identified several candidate genes associated with an increased risk of suicidal thoughts and behaviors and some of the notable findings are:

1. ESR1 (Estrogen Receptor 1): ESR1 has been previously identified as a causal genetic driver gene for PTSD and depression, both of which are risk factors for suicidal behaviors among veterans. Estrogen, which interacts with ESR1, is also suspected to play a role in sex differences in depression rates.[17]

2. DRD2 (Dopamine Receptor 2): DRD2 has been associated with suicide attempts, schizophrenia, mood disorders, ADHD, risky behaviors, and alcohol use disorder.

3. DCC (Deleted in Colorectal Cancer): DCC is expressed in brain tissue across the lifespan and has been linked to multiple psychiatric conditions. Elevated DCC levels have been observed in the brains of people who die by suicide.

4. TRAF3 (TNF Receptor-Associated Factor 3): TRAF3 is associated with antisocial behavior, substance use, and ADHD.[18]

Understanding the genetic underpinnings of suicidal thoughts is crucial for both individuals and mental health professionals. While genetic factors can increase vulnerability, they do not operate in

---

[17] https://psychiatry.duke.edu/news/four-genes-identified-heightening-risk-suicidal-thoughtsactions
[18] https://psychiatry.duke.edu/news/four-genes-identified-heightening-risk-suicidal-thoughtsactions

isolation. Environmental stressors, life experiences, and the broader context in which individuals live also contribute significantly to the emergence of suicidal thoughts.

This exploration emphasizes the importance of a holistic approach to mental health, considering both genetic and environmental factors. By acknowledging the role of genetics, individuals can be better equipped to engage in proactive mental health measures. Moreover, it underscores the necessity for comprehensive mental health care that addresses the unique intersection of genetic predispositions and life circumstances, fostering a landscape where individuals can navigate their mental well-being with resilience and understanding.

Suicidal thoughts are complex, and multiple factors often interact. Identifying and addressing these factors through professional help, therapy, and support systems is crucial in preventing and managing suicidal ideation. If you or someone you know is experiencing suicidal thoughts, seeking immediate assistance from mental health professionals or helplines is essential.

The Paths to Liberation from Suicidal Thoughts:
Seeking the guidance of mental health professionals forms a paramount path to liberation. Therapists, counselors, and psychiatrists possess the expertise to navigate the complexities of suicidal thoughts. Through tailored therapeutic approaches, individuals can unravel the underlying causes and develop coping mechanisms.

Immediate support is crucial in times of crisis. Accessing helplines or participating in support groups provides individuals with an outlet to express their emotions, receive empathetic understanding, and connect with others who have faced similar challenges.

In cases where mental health conditions contribute to suicidal thoughts, medication prescribed by a qualified healthcare professional can be instrumental. Properly managed medication can alleviate symptoms, stabilize mood, and create a foundation for further therapeutic work.

Developing a comprehensive safety plan is an empowering tool. This involves identifying triggers, establishing coping mechanisms, and creating a network of supportive individuals. A well-crafted safety plan serves as a proactive strategy to navigate moments of crisis.

Building a robust support system comprises friends, family, and loved ones who actively participate in an individual's well-being. Open communication, understanding, and empathy from this support network contribute significantly to the journey towards liberation.

Finding purpose and joy in life is pivotal. Engaging in activities that bring fulfillment, whether they are hobbies, volunteer work, or creative pursuits, can act as a powerful antidote to the darkness of suicidal thoughts.

Incorporating mindfulness and meditation into daily routines fosters self-awareness and resilience. These practices help individuals stay grounded in the present moment, manage stress, and develop a healthier perspective on challenges.

Educating friends and family about mental health challenges and suicidal thoughts is crucial. Creating an environment of understanding reduces stigma, encourages open communication, and strengthens the overall support system.

Remember, these paths to liberation are interconnected, forming a comprehensive approach to mental well-being. It is essential to tailor strategies to individual needs, acknowledging that everyone's journey towards liberation is unique. Professional guidance and a collaborative support system significantly enhance the effectiveness of these paths. Therefore, seeking professional help and compassionate support remains crucial for individuals experiencing suicidal thoughts.

THE METAMORPHOSIS OF THE MIND

Chapter 15

Strategies for Winning the Internal Wars

Understanding the Mind's Battlefield:
The mind's battlefield is the complex and dynamic arena where thoughts, emotions, and behaviors engage in a constant interplay. It represents the internal terrain where internal conflicts, self-doubt, and limiting beliefs emerge and manifest. This metaphorical battleground is where individuals grapple with their innermost struggles, facing challenges that impact their mental well-being.

In this context, the mind's battlefield encapsulates the various elements that contribute to the internal conflicts individuals experience. These may include negative thought patterns, self-critical tendencies, and emotional challenges. Understanding the intricacies of this mental landscape is crucial for developing effective strategies to navigate and overcome internal struggles.

The term emphasizes the need for self-awareness and intentional engagement in addressing the complexities of the mind. By recognizing the battlefield within, individuals can embark on a journey of self-discovery, resilience-building, and ultimately, victory over internal adversities.

Identification of Cognitive Patterns: The first step in the journey to conquer internal battles begins with a crucial step – the identification of cognitive patterns. This foundational process involves a deep exploration of the intricate landscape of the mind, where thoughts, emotions, and reactions intertwine. By undertaking this introspective journey, individuals actively engage in the examination of their mental habits, unveiling the underlying structures that shape their internal world.

The process of recognizing cognitive patterns is akin to peeling back the layers of a complex nature. It requires a keen awareness of one's thoughts and emotions, discerning recurring themes, and understanding the interplay between various elements of the mind. This introspective endeavor empowers individuals to become attuned to the nuances of their internal processes, shedding light on the intricate web of triggers and dynamics that contribute to internal conflicts.

Through this self-awareness, individuals not only gain valuable insights into the origins of their internal struggles but also lay the groundwork for transformative change. Identifying cognitive habits acts as a compass, guiding individuals toward a clearer understanding of the thought patterns that may fuel self-doubt, anxiety, or other challenges. Armed with this knowledge, they can navigate the complexities of their internal landscape with intentionality and purpose.

Awareness of Automatic Thoughts: Navigating the intricate terrain of the mind's battlefield demands a heightened awareness of automatic thoughts – those spontaneous and often insidious ideas that shape our perceptions and influence our emotional responses. Automatic thoughts, though fleeting, can wield considerable power in determining our outlook on ourselves, others, and the world.

In cultivating awareness of automatic thoughts, individuals embark on a journey of unraveling the complex web of cognitive processes. This involves closely observing the thoughts that spontaneously arise in response to situations, events, or even internal triggers. These automatic thoughts, often rooted in ingrained beliefs or past experiences, have the potential to shape our emotional landscape, contributing to feelings of self-doubt, anxiety, or inadequacy.

Understanding the genesis of automatic thoughts is a transformative process. It involves tracing the threads of these thoughts back to their origins and uncovering the influences that have shaped them over time. By recognizing the patterns and themes that characterize automatic thoughts, individuals gain a profound insight into the inner workings of their minds.

Armed with this awareness, individuals are empowered to challenge and redirect automatic thoughts that may be detrimental to their well-being. This deliberate and conscious engagement with one's cognitive processes fosters a sense of agency, allowing individuals to reshape their perceptions and, consequently, their emotional responses. In this way, awareness of automatic thoughts becomes a potent tool in the arsenal for winning internal wars and achieving mental resilience.

Cognitive Restructuring: Once negative thought patterns are identified, the next strategy involves challenging and restructuring them. This involves examining the evidence supporting these thoughts, exploring alternative perspectives, and replacing irrational beliefs with more balanced and constructive ones. Cognitive Restructuring emerges as a crucial strategy in the battle against negative thought patterns. Once these patterns are identified, the process involves a meticulous examination of the evidence that supports these thoughts. Individuals embark on a journey of exploration, seeking alternative perspectives that may offer a more balanced and constructive view of their experiences.

The heart of Cognitive Restructuring lies in the deliberate questioning of irrational beliefs. Individuals confront their negative thoughts with a critical eye, assessing their validity and accuracy. This process is akin to mental detective work, where individuals weigh the evidence supporting their automatic thoughts against the broader context of their experiences.

Through this intentional and methodical inquiry, individuals begin to unravel the distorted lens through which negative thoughts may have colored their perceptions. They discover that alternative viewpoints exist, ones that are grounded in a more balanced and realistic understanding of their circumstances.

As part of Cognitive Restructuring, individuals actively engage in the cultivation of new, positive beliefs to replace the irrational ones. This transformative process involves consciously choosing thoughts that are aligned with a healthier and more adaptive mindset. By actively participating in the reconstruction of their cognitive landscape, individuals pave the way for mental resilience and a more positive internal environment.

Building Emotional Intelligence: Enhancing emotional intelligence equips individuals with the capacity to navigate and understand their emotions. By recognizing, regulating, and expressing emotions effectively, individuals bolster their mental resilience in the face of internal challenges.

Building Emotional Intelligence emerges as a pivotal strategy in the quest for internal harmony. This strategy centers around the enhancement of individuals' capacity to navigate and comprehend their emotions more effectively. Emotional intelligence involves a multifaceted approach that encompasses the recognition, regulation, and expression of emotions in a manner that contributes to mental resilience.

At its core, this strategy encourages individuals to heighten their awareness of their emotional experiences. By fostering a keen recognition of various emotions as they arise, individuals lay the foundation for a deeper understanding of the intricate interplay between thoughts and feelings within the mind's landscape. This heightened awareness serves as a valuable tool for deciphering the emotional cues that may be intertwined with negative thought patterns.

Regulating emotions is the next crucial aspect of building emotional intelligence. This involves developing the ability to manage and modulate emotional responses, particularly in the face of challenging internal conflicts. Individuals learn to navigate the ebb and flow of emotions, cultivating a sense of balance and stability that acts as a buffer against the tumultuous currents of internal struggles.

Expressing emotions effectively forms the final pillar of this strategy. Through clear and constructive expression, individuals communicate their feelings in a manner that fosters understanding and connection. This skill not only enhances interpersonal relationships but also contributes to an internal environment where emotions are acknowledged and processed healthily.

In essence, Building Emotional Intelligence serves as a cornerstone for mental resilience. By honing the ability to recognize, regulate, and express emotions, individuals fortify their internal foundations, creating a more adaptive and robust mindset to confront the challenges of the mind's battlefield.

Stress Management Techniques: Developing effective stress management techniques is crucial for maintaining mental resilience. Strategies such as deep-breathing exercises, progressive muscle relaxation, and time-management skills empower individuals to navigate stressors more effectively.

The implementation of Stress Management Techniques emerges as a vital component in the arsenal of strategies aimed at fostering mental resilience. This strategy underscores the importance of developing effective tools to navigate and alleviate stressors that can impede internal harmony.

At its core, stress management involves the cultivation of various techniques designed to mitigate the impact of stress on mental well-being. Deep breathing exercises stand out as a fundamental approach, offering individuals a simple yet powerful method to regulate their physiological responses to stress. By focusing on intentional and controlled breathing patterns, individuals can activate the body's relaxation response, promoting a sense of calm amidst the storms of internal challenges.

Progressive Muscle Relaxation (PMR) represents another key stress management technique. This method involves systematically tensing and then relaxing different muscle groups, promoting physical and mental relaxation. By incorporating PMR into their routine, individuals can release tension stored in the body, creating a more tranquil internal environment.

Time-management skills play a crucial role in stress management, allowing individuals to organize and prioritize tasks effectively. The ability to allocate time efficiently reduces the likelihood of feeling overwhelmed, contributing to a more structured and manageable approach to daily challenges.

The overall goal of Stress Management Techniques is to empower individuals to face stressors with resilience and composure. By incorporating these strategies into their daily lives, individuals create a robust defense against the deleterious effects of stress on the mind's battlefield. This proactive approach not only enhances mental well-being but also equips individuals with the tools to navigate internal conflicts more adeptly.

Cultivating a Growth Mindset: Adopting a growth mindset involves viewing challenges as opportunities for learning and growth. Embracing setbacks as part of the journey fosters resilience and a positive outlook, counteracting the impact of internal conflicts.

The cultivation of a Growth Mindset emerges as a transformative strategy within the framework of winning internal wars. This approach centers on embracing challenges not as insurmountable obstacles but as fertile ground for learning and personal development.

At its core, a Growth Mindset involves a fundamental shift in perspective. Individuals with a growth mindset perceive setbacks, challenges, and failures as inherent components of the journey toward personal and intellectual growth. Instead of viewing difficulties as roadblocks, they see them as opportunities to learn, adapt, and strengthen their mental resilience.

This strategy encourages individuals to reframe their understanding of success and failure. Rather than perceiving failure as a definitive endpoint, a growth mindset interprets it as a temporary setback—one that provides valuable insights and lessons for future endeavors. This reframing not only diminishes the negative impact of internal conflicts but also cultivates a positive outlook on one's ability to navigate challenges and emerge stronger on the other side.

Embracing a Growth Mindset creates a foundation for continuous self-improvement and adaptability. It encourages individuals to approach internal conflicts with a sense of curiosity and a willingness to learn from the experience. By fostering resilience and a positive outlook, this strategy becomes a powerful tool in the pursuit of victory over the battles waged within the mind.

Seeking Social Support: Building a robust support network is a cornerstone of mental resilience. Sharing internal struggles with trusted friends, family, or mental health professionals provides perspectives, empathy, and a sense of connection that contributes to overall well-being.

The imperative of Seeking Social Support emerges as a pivotal strategy within the realm of winning internal wars. This strategy recognizes the intrinsic value of building a robust support network as a foundational element of mental resilience.

The importance of social connections cannot be overstated. Sharing internal struggles with trusted individuals, be they friends, family, or mental health professionals, serves as a powerful antidote to the isolation that internal conflicts can often induce. This open dialogue not only provides fresh perspectives but also fosters empathy, understanding, and a profound sense of connection.

The act of seeking social support contributes significantly to overall well-being. Engaging in meaningful conversations with individuals who offer support and understanding creates a network of emotional safety. Through these interactions, individuals gain valuable insights, diverse perspectives, and often, practical advice on navigating the complexities of their internal battles.

Trusted social connections serve as pillars of strength during challenging times, offering a source of encouragement, validation, and solace. The sharing of experiences and emotions within a supportive network creates a sense of community, mitigating the impact of isolation that often accompanies internal conflicts. This strategy, therefore, stands as a cornerstone in the arsenal of tools individuals can wield as they strive to conquer the internal wars waged within the recesses of the mind.

These strategies collectively form a comprehensive approach to winning internal wars. By understanding the mind's battlefield, challenging negative thought patterns, and cultivating mental resilience, individuals empower themselves to navigate internal conflicts with resilience, self-awareness, and the ability to foster positive change.

Chapter 16

The Metamorphosis Stages and Processes

The metamorphosis of the mind often begins with an awareness of existing thought patterns, beliefs, and cognitive processes. This recognition may be triggered by self-reflection, personal experiences, or exposure to new information.

The Stages of Metamorphosis:
The process often begins with introspection and self-reflection. Individuals may take a closer look at their thoughts, beliefs, and how they perceive the world. This self-awareness is crucial for identifying ingrained patterns.

Recognition may be prompted by specific events or experiences that create a sense of cognitive dissonance. This dissonance arises when there is a perceived inconsistency between one's beliefs and reality, leading to a discomfort that motivates individuals to reassess their cognitive framework.

Exposure to new and diverse information can be a catalyst for recognizing existing cognitive patterns. This can come from various sources such as books, articles, conversations, or experiences that challenge previously held beliefs.

Developing a capacity for critical thinking is integral to this stage. Individuals begin to question assumptions, challenge biases, and scrutinize the validity of their beliefs. This critical examination lays the groundwork for potential shifts in perspective.

Recognition involves an acknowledgment of cognitive biases that might influence one's thinking. Understanding that mental processes are not always objective but can be shaped by biases sets the stage for a more objective and open-minded approach to information.

The willingness to entertain the possibility that one's current beliefs might be subject to change is a characteristic of this stage. Open-mindedness fosters an environment where individuals can objectively assess their cognitive landscape.

Engaging in practices such as journaling or regular reflection can be instrumental. These activities provide a structured way for individuals to document their thoughts, emotions, and observations, facilitating a deeper understanding of their cognitive processes.

Journaling every day can offer a multitude of benefits that extend beyond just those pursuing a career in writing. Here are some reasons why daily writing can be advantageous for everyone:

Regular writing exercises your brain and enhances cognitive function. The process of putting thoughts into words helps reinforce neural connections, contributing to better memory retention.

The act of writing encourages individuals to explore a diverse range of words and expressions. This exploration naturally expands one's vocabulary, enabling clearer and more precise communication.

Writing regularly hones communication skills by forcing individuals to articulate their thoughts in a coherent and organized manner. This skill is transferable to various aspects of life, aiding in effective communication in both personal and professional settings.

Engaging in daily writing, whether it's a short story, blog post, or any other form of written expression, requires commitment. The decision to consistently allocate time to this activity fosters discipline and helps build habits that can be applied to other areas of life.

Like any other skill, writing is a craft that improves with practice. The more you write, the more you refine your style, structure, and overall storytelling abilities. This continuous development applies not only to professional writers but to anyone seeking self-improvement.

Writing regularly stimulates creativity by encouraging the exploration of ideas, perspectives, and imaginative scenarios, fostering a more creative mindset. This creativity can be beneficial in problem-solving and critical thinking.

Writing serves as a cathartic outlet for emotions and thoughts. It provides a structured means of expressing oneself, promoting self-awareness and emotional well-being.

In summary, journaling daily offers a wide array of cognitive, linguistic, and personal development benefits. It is a tool that can be utilized by individuals from all walks of life to enhance various aspects of their mental and emotional well-being.

The Processes of Metamorphosis:
As individuals become more aware of inconsistencies or conflicts between their existing beliefs and new information or experiences, they may experience cognitive dissonance. Cognitive dissonance is a psychological term for the discomfort that arises when there's a perceived inconsistency between one's beliefs and actions.

Cognitive dissonance is a psychological concept that refers to the discomfort or tension that arises when individuals hold conflicting beliefs, attitudes, or behaviors. In the context of the metamorphosis of the mind, cognitive dissonance catalyzes change by creating a noticeable misalignment between existing beliefs and new information or experiences. Here are the key elements of this stage:

Recognition of Inconsistencies: Individuals in the early stages of the metamorphosis become aware of inconsistencies between their current beliefs and the information or experiences they encounter. This recognition may result from encountering contradictory evidence, experiencing internal conflicts, or realizing that actions do not align with professed beliefs.

Cognitive dissonance triggers a sense of discomfort or unease. This discomfort arises from the internal conflict between conflicting beliefs or between beliefs and actions. Emotional responses such as anxiety, guilt, or confusion may accompany this discomfort.

The discomfort generated by cognitive dissonance motivates individuals to resolve the inconsistency. There is a natural inclination to seek harmony and alignment within one's belief system. This motivational aspect becomes a driving force for individuals to reevaluate and potentially adjust their existing cognitive framework.

Cognitive dissonance prompts individuals to critically reevaluate their beliefs. They may question the validity of long-held assumptions, challenge cognitive biases, and consider alternative perspectives that reconcile the conflicting elements.

Initially, individuals might resist acknowledging the inconsistencies, employing defense mechanisms to protect existing beliefs. This resistance is a natural response to the discomfort associated with cognitive dissonance. However, overcoming these defense mechanisms is crucial for the transformation to progress.

The resolution of cognitive dissonance involves seeking consistency within one's belief system. This can lead individuals to actively seek information that aligns with their existing beliefs or, conversely, to explore new perspectives that better align with their experiences.

Cognitive dissonance can result in behavioral changes as individuals strive to align their actions with their adjusted beliefs. This may involve making different choices, adopting new habits, or engaging in behaviors that better reflect the revised cognitive framework.

While cognitive dissonance can be uncomfortable, it is viewed as a valuable learning opportunity. It prompts individuals to confront the complexities of their beliefs and encourages a more nuanced understanding of the world.

As individuals navigate cognitive dissonance, it influences their decision-making processes. They may become more deliberate in evaluating information, considering alternative viewpoints, and making choices that align with their evolving beliefs.

Effectively addressing cognitive dissonance can be transformational. It opens the door to personal growth, expanded awareness, and a more adaptable and resilient mindset.

Openness to Change:
The metamorphosis process requires a certain degree of openness to change. Individuals must be willing to question their existing beliefs, challenge their assumptions, and consider alternative perspectives.

The third stage in the metamorphosis of the mind involves cultivating a mindset of openness to change. After recognizing existing thought patterns and experiencing cognitive dissonance, individuals must embrace a willingness to explore new ideas, perspectives, and ways of thinking. Here are the key details of this stage:

Openness to change requires a fundamental shift in mindset. Individuals move from a more rigid or fixed mindset to one that is flexible and adaptive. They acknowledge that change is a natural and potentially beneficial part of personal growth.

Openness is accompanied by a sense of curiosity and a desire for exploration. Individuals actively seek out new information, diverse viewpoints, and experiences that challenge or expand their existing understanding of the world.

Embracing openness involves a sense of humility. Individuals recognize that they may not have all the answers and that there is always room for learning and growth. This humility allows them to set aside ego-driven attachments to their current beliefs.

Open-minded individuals are ready to question their assumptions. They understand that assumptions, even long-held ones, can hinder personal development. This readiness to question leads to a deeper and more nuanced exploration of ideas.

Openness is closely linked to adaptability. Individuals who are open to change are better equipped to adapt to new information and evolving circumstances. They view change as an opportunity for learning rather than a threat to their existing worldview.

Openness requires emotional resilience. It involves facing uncertainty, confronting cognitive dissonance, and navigating the discomfort that may arise from challenging one's own beliefs. Emotional resilience allows individuals to persevere through this process.

An open mindset involves an acceptance of the complexity inherent in the world. Instead of seeking overly simplistic explanations, individuals are comfortable with ambiguity and recognize that reality often exists in shades of gray.

Openness is associated with empathy. As individuals explore new perspectives, they develop a greater understanding and empathy for the experiences and viewpoints of others. This empathetic awareness contributes to more compassionate interactions.

Openness involves developing a tolerance for ambiguity. It means being comfortable with the idea that not everything has a clear-cut answer, and that uncertainty is a natural part of the learning and growth process.

Embracing openness leads to an expansion of one's worldview. Individuals begin to see the world through a broader lens, incorporating diverse perspectives, cultural nuances, and a deeper appreciation for the complexity of human experience.

Open-minded individuals are often more inclined to engage in collaborative learning. They value the exchange of ideas, appreciate diverse contributions, and recognize that collective wisdom can lead to richer insights.

The openness to change is often driven by intrinsic motivation. Individuals are internally motivated by a genuine desire for personal growth, learning, and a more comprehensive understanding of themselves and the world.

In summary, openness to change is a pivotal stage in the metamorphosis of the mind. It involves a shift in mindset, a curiosity for exploration, a readiness to question assumptions, and the development of emotional resilience. This openness sets the stage for transformative growth and an enriched perspective on life.

Exploration and Learning:
Individuals undergoing a metamorphosis of the mind often engage in active exploration and learning. This may involve reading diverse perspectives, seeking out new experiences, or engaging in conversations with people who hold different views.

The fourth stage in the metamorphosis of the mind centers around active exploration and continuous learning. Following the recognition of existing thought patterns, cognitive dissonance, and an openness to change, individuals engage in intentional efforts to broaden their knowledge, challenge assumptions, and deepen their understanding of themselves and the world. Here are the key details of this stage:

Individuals in this stage actively seek out new information, diverse perspectives, and a range of experiences. This may involve reading books, articles, and research, attending lectures, participating in discussions, or exploring various forms of media to gain exposure to different viewpoints.

Exploration involves a deliberate effort to expose oneself to a diversity of perspectives. This may include engaging with viewpoints that challenge one's existing beliefs, fostering a more comprehensive and nuanced understanding of various subjects.

Exploration is accompanied by the development of critical thinking skills. Individuals learn to critically evaluate information, discern between reliable and unreliable sources, and analyze arguments and evidence. This skill set is crucial for forming well-informed opinions.

Learning is not confined to theoretical knowledge but extends to experiential learning. Individuals actively seek out new experiences that provide practical insights and contribute to personal growth. These experiences could include travel, volunteering, or taking on new challenges.

A key characteristic of this stage is the maintenance of continuous curiosity. Individuals adopt a mindset that views every encounter as an opportunity to learn. This curiosity becomes a driving force for ongoing exploration and intellectual curiosity.

Exploration is not only about acquiring knowledge but also about cultivating practical skills. Individuals may seek to develop skills that align with their evolving interests and contribute to their personal and professional development.

Growth often occurs outside of one's comfort zone. In this stage, individuals intentionally seek out challenges that push them beyond familiar boundaries. This could involve tackling difficult subjects, engaging in debates, or taking on responsibilities that foster personal and intellectual growth.

Recognizing the interconnectedness of knowledge, individuals may engage in interdisciplinary learning. This involves exploring topics that span multiple disciplines, fostering a holistic understanding of complex issues.

Learning is not limited to individual efforts. Individuals in this stage recognize the value of networking and collaboration. They engage with diverse communities, fostering opportunities for shared learning and collaborative exploration.

Through exploration, individuals develop the ability to adapt to new perspectives. They learn to appreciate differing viewpoints without necessarily adopting them, enhancing their capacity for empathy and understanding.

The goal of exploration is not just the accumulation of information but the integration of learning into one's existing knowledge base. This integration contributes to a more coherent and comprehensive mental framework.

Individuals may set specific goals for their learning journey. These goals could be short-term or long-term, aligning with personal aspirations, career objectives, or broader interests.

In summary, the stage of exploration and learning is characterized by active engagement with new information, diverse perspectives, and experiential learning. It involves continuous curiosity, critical thinking, and the intentional cultivation of skills, contributing to a transformative and dynamic process of intellectual and personal development.

Shift in Perspective:
A significant aspect of the metamorphosis is the actual shift in perspective. This can involve a re-evaluation of one's values, beliefs, priorities, and even the way they perceive the world and

themselves. It's a transformative process that can lead to a more nuanced and complex understanding of various aspects of life.

The fifth stage in the metamorphosis of the mind involves a substantive shift in perspective. Building on the foundation of recognition, cognitive dissonance, openness to change, and exploration, individuals undergo a transformative change in the way they perceive themselves, others, and the world. Here are the key details of this stage:

A significant aspect of the shift in perspective is the re-evaluation of core beliefs. Individuals question deeply ingrained beliefs that may have shaped their identity and influenced their decision-making. This process often requires a high level of introspection and a willingness to challenge long-standing assumptions.

The shift in perspective represents a paradigm shift, wherein individuals move away from conventional or limiting frameworks of thinking. This may involve questioning societal norms, cultural expectations, or personal ideologies that were previously unquestioned.

As perspectives shift, there is an expansion of consciousness. Individuals begin to see the world through a broader lens, considering multiple viewpoints and embracing the idea that there are diverse ways of interpreting reality. This expanded consciousness contributes to a more inclusive and holistic understanding.

The shift in perspective often involves recognizing the interconnectedness of all things. Individuals grasp the intricate web of relationships between themselves, others, and the world. This interconnected perspective fosters a sense of responsibility and empathy for the well-being of the broader community.

Individuals become more accepting of the fact that not everything can be neatly categorized or understood. This acceptance of ambiguity allows for a more nuanced and sophisticated worldview.

There is an appreciation for the complexity of human experience and the multifaceted nature of issues. Rather than seeking oversimplified explanations, individuals acknowledge the intricate layers that contribute to the richness and diversity of life.

The shift in perspective often leads to a re-evaluation of personal values. Individuals may prioritize values that align more closely with their evolving understanding of the world. This could involve a greater emphasis on compassion, social justice, environmental consciousness, or other values that reflect a deeper awareness.

Individuals develop cognitive flexibility, allowing them to adapt their thinking to different situations and challenges. This flexibility enables a more adaptive and resilient approach to navigating the complexities of life.

The shift in perspective can profoundly impact one's self-identity. Individuals may experience a transformation in how they define themselves, moving away from rigid or limiting self-concepts toward a more fluid and evolving sense of identity.

Transformed individuals actively seek to integrate diverse perspectives into their understanding. They appreciate the value of hearing different voices, acknowledging cultural diversity, and recognizing the richness that emerges from the coexistence of varied perspectives.

The shift in perspective often involves aligning with a more authentic and personally resonant truth. Individuals may discover a truer version of themselves that is less influenced by external expectations and more guided by an internal compass.

A transformed perspective positively impacts relationships. Individuals become more open to understanding the perspectives of others, fostering empathy, and cultivating meaningful connections built on shared values and mutual respect.

The shift in perspective extends to emotional and spiritual dimensions. Individuals may experience heightened emotional intelligence, a deeper connection to their spiritual beliefs, and a sense of inner peace that comes from aligning with a more authentic understanding of themselves and the world.

In summary, the shift in perspective is a profound stage in the metamorphosis of the mind. It involves reevaluating core beliefs, expanding consciousness, embracing ambiguity, and aligning with values that reflect a more authentic and nuanced understanding of the self and the world. This transformative shift lays the groundwork for continued personal and intellectual growth.

Development of Empathy:
As the mind undergoes a metamorphosis, individuals may develop a deeper sense of empathy and understanding toward others. This

involves recognizing and appreciating diverse experiences, backgrounds, and perspectives.

The sixth stage in the metamorphosis of the mind involves the development of empathy. As individuals undergo a shift in perspective and deepen their understanding of diverse experiences, the capacity for empathy expands. Empathy is the ability to understand and share the feelings of another. This stage is crucial for fostering meaningful connections, promoting social harmony, and contributing to a more compassionate worldview.

Here are the key details of this stage:
Cognitive empathy is the intellectual understanding of another person's perspective, emotions, or experiences. It involves the ability to "put oneself in someone else's shoes" and grasp their point of view. Individuals in this stage actively seek to understand the thoughts and emotions of others, even if they differ from their own.

Affective empathy goes beyond intellectual understanding; it involves an emotional resonance with the feelings of others. Individuals develop a heightened sensitivity to the emotional experiences of those around them. This emotional attunement allows for a deeper connection and a more profound sense of shared humanity.

Empathy is demonstrated through empathic listening—a skill where individuals genuinely listen to others without judgment, interruption, or preconceived notions. This type of listening fosters trust and creates a supportive environment for open communication.

Empathy involves recognizing and appreciating the diversity of human experiences. Individuals in this stage understand that each person's background, cultural context, and life circumstances contribute to a unique set of challenges and perspectives.

Developing empathy requires a conscious effort to overcome stereotypes and prejudices. Individuals challenge preconceived notions and actively work to understand individuals beyond superficial characteristics, fostering a more inclusive and tolerant mindset.

Empathy is not passive; it often translates into compassionate action. Individuals in this stage are more inclined to take actions that contribute to the well-being of others. This could involve acts of kindness, advocacy for social justice, or involvement in community initiatives.

Empathy strengthens interpersonal connections. Individuals become attuned to the emotions of those around them, creating a more supportive and connected social environment. This sense of connection enhances the quality of relationships and contributes to overall well-being.

Empathy fosters a deep respect for diverse perspectives. Even when individuals do not agree with others, they can appreciate the validity of different viewpoints. This respect contributes to constructive dialogue and collaboration in various personal and professional contexts.

The development of empathy often leads to a reduction in interpersonal conflict. When individuals understand and empathize with each other's perspectives, there is a greater likelihood of finding common ground and resolving differences through communication and understanding.

Empathy extends beyond individual relationships to encompass a global perspective. Individuals in this stage recognize the interconnectedness of the world and empathize with the challenges faced by individuals and communities on a broader scale.

Empathy is closely linked to a commitment to social justice. Individuals may become advocates for marginalized groups, actively working to address systemic inequalities and contribute to a more just and equitable society.

The development of empathy is a key component of emotional intelligence. Individuals with high emotional intelligence navigate social interactions with greater sensitivity, understanding, and emotional regulation.

As individuals develop empathy, they may also contribute to nurturing empathy in others. By modeling empathic behavior and promoting empathy in social and educational settings, they contribute to the cultivation of a more compassionate society.

In summary, the development of empathy is a transformative stage in the metamorphosis of the mind. It involves cognitive and affective dimensions, fostering a deeper understanding of others, promoting interpersonal connection, and contributing to positive social change. Empathy becomes a guiding principle in navigating the complexities of human relationships and promoting a more compassionate and understanding world.

Re-evaluation of Goals and Priorities:
The transformation may prompt individuals to reevaluate their life goals, priorities, and what they find meaningful. This can lead to a realignment of personal and professional aspirations.

The seventh stage in the metamorphosis of the mind involves a thoughtful re-evaluation of personal goals and priorities. As individuals undergo shifts in perspective, develop empathy, and gain a deeper understanding of themselves and the world, they may find it necessary to reassess their aspirations and the values that guide their lives. Here are the key details of this stage:

Individuals engage in reflective self-examination to assess their current goals and priorities. This involves considering whether these goals align with their evolving beliefs, values, and the broader perspective gained through the metamorphosis process.

The re-evaluation process centers around aligning goals with personal values. Individuals question whether their current goals are in harmony with the principles and values that have emerged or evolved during their transformative journey.

The re-evaluation stage prompts individuals to clarify their core values. This includes identifying the principles that are most important to them, such as integrity, compassion, justice, personal growth, or contribution to society.

As goals are reassessed, there may be a shift in life purpose. Individuals contemplate whether their current life trajectory serves a meaningful purpose that aligns with their deeper understanding of self and the world.

The re-evaluation often involves a prioritization of overall well-being. Individuals may reconsider whether their goals contribute positively to their mental, emotional, and physical health, as well as to the well-being of those around them.

Individuals explore the integration of personal and professional aspects of their lives. The re-evaluation process considers whether there is alignment between personal values and the values embedded in their chosen career or life path.

The stage of re-evaluation requires individuals to balance short-term and long-term goals. They consider whether their current pursuits contribute to both immediate objectives and the broader, more enduring goals that shape their life journey.

The re-evaluation process may lead individuals to explore new passions or areas of interest. As they gain a clearer sense of their values and priorities, they may discover previously overlooked or undiscovered areas that align more closely with their authentic selves.

Individuals assess their relationship with materialism and external markers of success. The re-evaluation involves questioning whether material pursuits and external validations align with a more authentic and personally meaningful definition of success.

Goals are reevaluated in the context of their environmental and social impact. Individuals consider whether their pursuits contribute positively to the community, society, or the broader world, reflecting a sense of social responsibility.

The re-evaluation of goals reflects an adaptability to change. Individuals recognize that life is dynamic, and as they grow and evolve, their goals and priorities may need to adjust accordingly. This adaptability allows for continued alignment with personal values.

The criteria for decision-making evolve during this stage. Individuals may shift from purely outcome-based decision-making to a more process-oriented approach that considers how their choices align with their values and contribute to their overall sense of fulfillment.

The re-evaluation stage encourages mindful goal setting. Individuals set goals with greater intentionality, ensuring that each goal contributes positively to their overall sense of purpose, well-being, and fulfillment.

The ultimate aim of reevaluating goals and priorities is to strive for authenticity. Individuals seek a congruence between their external actions and their internal beliefs, cultivating a life that is true to themselves and their evolving understanding of what truly matters.

In summary, the re-evaluation of goals and priorities is a pivotal stage in the metamorphosis of the mind. It involves a thoughtful examination of one's life direction, aligning goals with personal values, and striving for authenticity in both personal and professional pursuits. This stage contributes to a more intentional and fulfilling life path shaped by a deep understanding of the self and the world.

Enhanced Self-Awareness:
Metamorphosis often results in enhanced self-awareness. Individuals may gain a clearer understanding of their thought processes, motivations, and the factors that influence their decision-making.

The eighth stage in the metamorphosis of the mind involves the enhancement of self-awareness. As individuals progress through the transformative journey, engage in reflective practices, and reevaluate their goals and priorities, they experience a deepening awareness of their thoughts, emotions, motivations, and behaviors. Here are the key details of this stage:

Enhanced self-awareness begins with intentional introspection and reflection. Individuals dedicate time to observe their thoughts, emotions, and actions. This self-reflective process allows for a deeper understanding of the underlying factors shaping their behavior.

Through self-awareness, individuals identify recurring patterns in their thoughts and behaviors. This includes recognizing habits, automatic responses, and cognitive biases that may have been previously overlooked. Awareness of these patterns is essential for personal growth and change.

Enhanced self-awareness is a cornerstone of emotional intelligence. Individuals develop a heightened sensitivity to their own emotions and the ability to navigate and regulate these emotions effectively.

This contributes to improved interpersonal relationships and decision-making.

Self-awareness involves accepting one's imperfections and vulnerabilities. Being self-aware does not imply perfection but rather an acknowledgment of the multifaceted nature of the self. This acceptance fosters self-compassion and resilience.

The process of self-awareness clarifies personal values and beliefs. Individuals gain insight into the principles that guide their lives, helping them make decisions that align with their authentic selves. This clarity provides a strong foundation for intentional living.

Self-aware individuals practice mindful living. They bring conscious awareness to their daily activities, interactions, and experiences. This mindfulness cultivates a deeper appreciation for the present moment and a more intentional approach to life.

Enhanced self-awareness allows individuals to identify their triggers—events or situations that evoke strong emotional responses. Recognizing these triggers provides an opportunity for proactive management, leading to healthier emotional reactions.

Individuals explore their motivations, gaining insight into the driving forces behind their goals and actions. This understanding helps them align their pursuits with authentic and meaningful aspirations.

Self-awareness facilitates alignment with one's authentic self. Individuals become more attuned to their true desires, passions, and values, enabling them to lead lives that resonate with their core identity.

Self-aware individuals are open to receiving feedback from others. They recognize the value of external perspectives in furthering their understanding of themselves. Constructive feedback becomes a tool for continuous growth.

Enhanced self-awareness contributes to the cultivation of empathy towards others. Understanding one's struggles and vulnerabilities fosters a compassionate and empathetic approach to the challenges faced by others.

Self-aware individuals demonstrate adaptability and flexibility in the face of change. They are better equipped to navigate challenges, as they understand their strengths and limitations, allowing for more effective problem-solving.

Self-awareness positively influences decision-making. Individuals are more conscious of their values and priorities, enabling them to make choices that align with their long-term goals and overall well-being.

Self-awareness is linked to a growth mindset—an understanding that personal qualities can be developed through effort and learning. Individuals embrace challenges, view failures as opportunities for growth, and persist in the face of setbacks.

Enhanced self-awareness is associated with improved mental health. Individuals are better equipped to manage stress, anxiety, and other emotional challenges, fostering a sense of resilience and overall psychological well-being.

In summary, enhanced self-awareness is a fundamental stage in the metamorphosis of the mind. It involves introspection, identification of patterns, acceptance of imperfections, clarification of values, and mindful living. This deepened awareness of oneself contributes to personal growth, emotional intelligence, and the ability to lead a more intentional and fulfilling life.

Integration of New Beliefs:
The transformation involves integrating new beliefs and perspectives into one's cognitive framework. This doesn't necessarily mean abandoning one's previous beliefs entirely but rather synthesizing new information with existing knowledge.

The ninth stage in the metamorphosis of the mind involves the integration of the transformative experiences, insights, and self-awareness gained throughout the journey. At this stage, individuals strive to create a holistic understanding of themselves, unifying various aspects of their identity, beliefs, and values into a cohesive and authentic whole. Here are the key details of this stage:

Integration involves synthesizing the diverse experiences encountered during the transformative journey. Individuals reflect on how each stage, realization, and challenge contributed to their growth and understanding. This synthesis fosters a sense of coherence in their life narrative.

At this stage, individuals work towards creating a unified self-concept. This means integrating various facets of their identity, including personal values, beliefs, strengths, vulnerabilities, and passions. The goal is to form a more comprehensive and authentic understanding of who they are.

The integration process emphasizes aligning one's life choices and actions with core values. Individuals strive to live by their deeply held principles, fostering a sense of integrity and authenticity in their endeavors.

Individuals in this stage navigate the delicate balance between personal aspirations and external expectations. They consciously choose paths that align with their authentic selves while acknowledging and managing societal, familial, or cultural expectations.

Emotional experiences are integrated into the overall understanding of self. This includes acknowledging and accepting a wide range of emotions, understanding their origins, and developing healthy ways to express and regulate them. Emotional integration contributes to emotional intelligence and resilience.

Integration extends to the mind-body connection. Individuals recognize the interconnectedness of mental and physical well-being. Practices such as mindfulness, exercise, and nutrition are embraced as integral components of holistic health.

The integrated self embraces complexity. Individuals acknowledge that they are multifaceted beings with layers of experiences, beliefs, and emotions. This acceptance allows for a more nuanced and compassionate understanding of oneself.

The integration stage often involves cultivating gratitude for the journey and the lessons learned. Individuals appreciate the challenges, successes, and even the setbacks, recognizing that each contributes to their growth and development.

Through integration, individuals develop a life philosophy—a set of guiding principles that inform their choices, relationships, and overall approach to life. This philosophy serves as a compass for navigating future challenges and decisions.

Integration includes a deepened connection with others. Individuals appreciate the shared human experience, recognizing the common threads that connect people. This sense of connection fosters empathy, compassion, and a collaborative mindset.

The integrated self remains open to continued learning and adaptation. Individuals understand that growth is an ongoing process, and they approach life with curiosity and a willingness to evolve in response to new experiences and insights.

Integration leads to personal leadership—an ability to guide one's own life with purpose and authenticity. Individuals become the leaders of their journeys, making choices aligned with their values and contributing positively to the world around them.

The ultimate goal of integration is holistic well-being. Individuals seek well-being not only in specific areas of life but as a holistic concept encompassing physical, emotional, social, and spiritual dimensions. This approach promotes a balanced and fulfilling life.

Integrated individuals authentically express themselves in various aspects of life—relationships, work, creative pursuits, and personal growth. This authenticity is characterized by a genuine alignment between inner values and outward actions.

Integrated individuals often find fulfillment in contributing to the well-being of others and society. This may involve sharing insights, mentoring, or actively participating in initiatives that align with their values and contribute to positive social change.

In summary, the stage of integration and holistic self marks the culmination of the metamorphosis of the mind. It involves synthesizing experiences, aligning with core values, balancing expectations, and fostering a unified and authentic self. Integrated individuals navigate life with purpose, resilience, and a deep sense of well-being.

Continuous Growth:
The metamorphosis of the mind is not a one-time event but an ongoing process of growth and development. Individuals who experience this transformation are often more open to continued learning, adaptability, and evolving perspectives.

The tenth and final stage in the metamorphosis of the mind is characterized by a commitment to ongoing growth and evolution. This stage reflects the understanding that personal development is a continuous journey rather than a destination. Individuals in this stage embrace change, cultivate a growth mindset, and remain open to new experiences and insights. Here are the key details of this stage:

Ongoing growth involves a commitment to lifelong learning. Individuals recognize that knowledge is dynamic, and there is always more to discover. They actively seek out learning opportunities, whether through formal education, self-directed study, or experiential learning.

Individuals in this stage exhibit a high degree of adaptability. They embrace change as a natural part of life and are resilient in the face of challenges. This adaptability allows them to navigate the complexities of an ever-changing world with a sense of curiosity and flexibility.

Rather than avoiding challenges, individuals committed to ongoing growth actively seek them out. Challenges are viewed as opportunities for learning and development. They understand that facing difficulties can lead to personal resilience and expanded capabilities.

Ongoing growth involves the refinement of existing skills and the acquisition of new ones. Individuals continually strive to improve their abilities, whether in their professional field, personal interests, or interpersonal skills. This commitment to skill development contributes to a sense of mastery.

Reflective practices become a habitual part of the ongoing growth process. Individuals regularly take time for introspection, assessing their progress, identifying areas for improvement, and celebrating achievements. This self-reflection serves as a compass for their continued development.

Individuals with a growth mindset believe that their abilities and intelligence can be developed with effort and learning. They see challenges as opportunities to grow, and setbacks as valuable learning experiences. Cultivating a growth mindset is a key aspect of ongoing personal evolution.

Those committed to ongoing growth set stretch goals that challenge their existing capabilities. These goals go beyond the comfort zone, encouraging individuals to reach new heights and expand their horizons. The pursuit of stretch goals fuels continuous improvement.

Networking and collaborative learning remain integral to ongoing growth. Individuals seek out diverse perspectives, engage in meaningful conversations, and collaborate with others to exchange ideas and insights. Networking contributes to a broader understanding of the world and fosters a sense of community.

Ongoing growth encompasses a commitment to physical, mental, and emotional well-being. Individuals prioritize self-care practices, healthy lifestyle choices, and activities that contribute to overall wellness. A holistic approach to well-being supports sustained personal development.

Resilience is a key attribute in the ongoing growth journey. Individuals learn from setbacks, bounce back from challenges, and use adversity as a catalyst for personal development. The cultivation of resilience ensures a robust and adaptive approach to life's ups and downs.

Individuals engaged in ongoing growth often seek mentorship and may also take on mentorship roles themselves. Mentorship provides guidance, encouragement, and the sharing of wisdom between individuals at different stages of their journeys. It fosters a sense of community and mutual support.

Ongoing growth extends to contributing to the well-being of others. Individuals actively look for ways to share their knowledge, experiences, and resources to positively impact the lives of those around them. Contribution becomes a meaningful aspect of their ongoing journey.

Individuals in this stage remain open to new perspectives. They actively seek out diverse viewpoints, challenge their assumptions, and remain curious about the world. This ongoing exploration contributes to a rich and multifaceted understanding of life.

As values continue to evolve, individuals in this stage regularly assess their alignment with these values. They make conscious choices that reflect their evolving principles and contribute to a sense of authenticity and purpose.

Celebrating achievements, both big and small, is an important aspect of ongoing growth. Individuals acknowledge and appreciate their progress, fostering a positive and motivated mindset for the continued journey ahead.

Those committed to ongoing growth consider the legacy they want to leave and the impact they want to have on the world. They actively shape their contributions to create a positive and lasting influence on future generations.

In summary, the stage of ongoing growth and evolution encapsulates a mindset of continuous learning, adaptability, resilience, and a commitment to personal and collective well-being. It reflects a dynamic and purposeful approach to life, where each day is seen as an opportunity for further development and a positive contribution to the world.

Impact on Behavior:
The changes in the mind are likely to manifest in one's behavior. This could involve changes in decision-making, communication, relationships, and overall lifestyle choices.

A transformed mind brings heightened consciousness to decision-making. Individuals become more aware of their values, goals, and the potential consequences of their choices. Decisions are more likely to align with the individual's core values, reflecting a deeper understanding of what truly matters to them.

The mind's metamorphosis encourages a shift from short-term thinking to consideration of the long-term impact of decisions, fostering a more sustainable approach. A transformed mind often leads to enhanced empathy, influencing the way individuals communicate. There is a greater ability to understand and connect with others on an emotional level.

The clarity gained through self-awareness allows for more articulate and authentic expression of ideas, thoughts, and feelings. Transformed individuals engage in active listening, valuing others' perspectives and fostering meaningful dialogue.

THE METAMORPHOSIS OF THE MIND

Changes in the mind contribute to deeper and more meaningful connections with others. Authenticity and vulnerability become integral to building and sustaining relationships. Transformed minds often exhibit a heightened respect for diversity in relationships, embracing differences and valuing the uniqueness of everyone.

The metamorphosis facilitates improved conflict resolution skills, with a focus on understanding, empathy, and collaborative problem-solving. Mindful Living: Transformed minds promote mindful living, encouraging individuals to be fully present in their daily experiences and appreciate the richness of each moment.

Alignment with Well-Being: Lifestyle choices are aligned with overall well-being, encompassing physical, mental, and emotional health. Self-care practices become integral to the daily routine. Individuals with transformed minds often pursue activities and endeavors that align with their passions and contribute to a sense of purpose. A transformed mind enhances adaptability, allowing individuals to navigate unexpected challenges with resilience and flexibility.

The metamorphosis fosters an openness to change, encouraging individuals to embrace new opportunities and experiences for personal and professional growth. Commitment to Learning: Transformed minds are characterized by a continuous commitment to learning and personal growth. Individuals actively seek out opportunities for self-improvement.

The changes in the mind facilitate more intentional goal setting, and the individual is better equipped to achieve these goals through focused effort and determination. Contributions to Others: Individuals with transformed minds often seek to positively impact their communities and society at large. They may engage in volunteer work, advocacy, or other initiatives aligned with their values.

The changes in behavior extend to a commitment to promoting positive change in the world, whether on a small scale in personal relationships or on a larger scale in societal structures. Enhanced Emotional Intelligence: The metamorphosis contributes to enhanced emotional intelligence, allowing individuals to understand, manage, and express emotions healthily and constructively.

Individuals who have undergone a metamorphosis of the mind may develop greater resilience to change and ambiguity. The ability to adapt to new information and experiences becomes a valuable aspect of their cognitive and emotional resilience.

The metamorphosis of the mind often bestows individuals with an enhanced resilience to change and ambiguity. This resilience, observed in both cognitive and emotional domains, becomes a valuable asset as individuals navigate the complexities of life.

THE METAMORPHOSIS OF THE MIND

Chapter 17

Five Keys to Boosting Your Mind

1. *The Power of Wholesome Music*:
Music has a powerful impact on the human mind and can act as a stimulus. The ability of music to evoke emotions and memories makes it a unique form of communication that transcends linguistic and cultural barriers.

Studies have shown that music can activate various parts of the brain, including the emotional centers, which are responsible for regulating our moods and emotions.[19] The beat, rhythm, melody, and lyrics of a piece of music can stimulate different regions of the brain, leading to the release of neurotransmitters such as dopamine, which is associated with pleasure and reward.

Music can also affect the brain's temporal lobe, which is responsible for processing sensory information and regulating our attention. This explains why music can be so captivating and can command our attention even when we are not consciously paying attention to it.

---

[19] https://webmedy.com/blog/music-brain/

The power of music to stimulate and boost the human mind is due to its unique ability to activate various regions of the brain, leading to the release of neurotransmitters and the evocation of emotions and memories.

Music stimulates several parts of the brain, including the auditory cortex, which is responsible for processing sound, and the limbic system, which is associated with emotions and memories.[20]

Additionally, music can activate the motor cortex, which is involved in movement and coordination. This stimulation occurs as the brain processes the musical sounds and rhythm, and can result in changes in mood, attention, and perception. The exact way in which music stimulates the brain is still being studied by researchers, but it is believed to involve the release of neurotransmitters, such as dopamine, and the creation of neural networks that are strengthened with repeated exposure to music.[21]

Music has a powerful impact on the brain, influencing emotions, memories, and even physical responses. When we listen to music, different parts of the brain are activated, and the brain processes the sound, rhythm, and melody in a way that can have a profound effect on our state of mind and overall well-being.

The auditory cortex, located in the temporal lobe of the brain, is responsible for processing sound and plays a key role in our

---

[20]https://www.health.harvard.edu/mind-and-mood/music-can-boost-memory-and-mood
[21]https://www.medicaldaily.com/your-brain-music-how-our-brains-process-melodies-pull-our-heartstrings-271007

perception of music. This area of the brain is activated when we listen to music, allowing us to recognize patterns and structure in the sound.

The limbic system, which includes the amygdala and hippocampus, is associated with emotions and memories. Music has been shown to activate this system, leading to changes in mood and the formation of emotional connections to specific songs or pieces of music.

The motor cortex, which is involved in movement and coordination, is also activated by music, particularly when we tap our feet or dance to a beat. This connection between music and physical movement is thought to be due to the relationship between music and rhythm.

The exact way in which music affects the brain is still being studied by researchers, but it is thought to involve the release of neurotransmitters, such as dopamine, which are associated with pleasure and reward. Additionally, repeated exposure to music can lead to the creation of neural networks that are strengthened over time, allowing us to recall memories and emotions that are associated with specific songs or pieces of music.

Overall, music has a complex and multi-faceted impact on the brain, and its effects are the result of the interaction between several different brain systems.

Autosuggestion
Oral suggestion or auto-suggestion is a method of influencing the subconscious mind through repeated verbal affirmations. The idea

behind autosuggestion is that by repeatedly telling yourself positive statements, you can change your beliefs and attitudes and influence your behavior.

Auto-suggestion works by bypassing the critical conscious mind and accessing the subconscious mind, which is thought to be more susceptible to suggestion. When a person repeatedly hears a suggestion, it becomes embedded in their subconscious and can influence their thoughts, feelings, and actions.

Auto-suggestion has been used for a variety of purposes, including changing negative self-talk, increasing motivation, reducing stress and anxiety, and improving sleep. It is often used as a self-help tool and is sometimes incorporated into other techniques such as meditation and visualization.

The effectiveness of autosuggestion depends on several factors, including the frequency and consistency of the suggestions, the strength of the person's belief in the suggestion, and the compatibility of the suggestion with their values and goals. To be effective, suggestions must be clear, specific, and positive, and must be repeated regularly.

Oral suggestion or auto-suggestion can stimulate and influence the human mind by providing positive, repeated affirmations that access the subconscious mind and change beliefs, attitudes, and behaviors.

Oral suggestion or auto-suggestion is a powerful tool for personal change and improvement that operates by influencing the subconscious mind. The concept of autosuggestion is based on the idea that by repeatedly telling yourself positive affirmations, you can change your beliefs, attitudes, and behaviors and influence your thoughts, emotions, and experiences.

The subconscious mind is thought to be more susceptible to suggestion than the conscious mind, which is responsible for critical thinking and analysis. By bypassing the conscious mind, oral suggestion or auto-suggestion can have a direct and lasting impact on the subconscious, leading to changes in attitudes, beliefs, and behaviors.

Auto-suggestion can be used for a wide range of purposes, from overcoming negative self-talk and increasing self-confidence, to reducing stress and anxiety, improving sleep, and increasing motivation. To be effective, suggestions should be repeated regularly and consistently and should be clear, specific, and positive.

It is also important to ensure that the suggestions are compatible with the person's values, goals, and beliefs. The more a person believes in the suggestion, the more likely they are to experience positive results.

Auto-suggestion can be done in several ways, including verbal affirmations, writing positive statements, or repeating affirmations in the mind. It is often combined with other techniques such as visualization, meditation, and affirmations, to increase its effectiveness.

In conclusion, oral suggestion or auto-suggestion is a simple but powerful tool that can be used to stimulate and influence the human mind. Providing repeated positive affirmations, can change beliefs, attitudes, and behaviors and lead to lasting personal growth and improvement.

Getting enough sleep:
A good night's sleep is essential for optimal brain function. Lack of sleep can lead to decreased focus, decreased motivation, and impaired decision-making.

Getting enough quality sleep is crucial for optimal brain function and overall health. Sleep plays an important role in the consolidation of memories, allowing the brain to process and store information from the day. In addition, sleep helps to boost focus and concentration, which are important for learning and problem-solving.[22]

When a person lacks sleep, their ability to concentrate, make decisions, and recall information is significantly impacted. This can result in decreased motivation, impaired decision-making, and increased stress and anxiety. Over time, chronic sleep deprivation can lead to more serious health problems, including obesity, heart disease, and depression.[23]

To boost the brain and support overall health, it's important to get enough quality sleep each night. The National Sleep Foundation recommends 7-9 hours of sleep per night for adults.[24] To improve the quality of sleep, individuals can establish a bedtime routine,

---

[22] https://www.sleepfoundation.org/how-sleep-works/benefits-of-sleep
[23] https://newsinhealth.nih.gov/2021/04/good-sleep-good-health
[24] https://pubmed.ncbi.nlm.nih.gov/29073398/

avoid screens for at least an hour before bed, and create a sleep-conducive environment by keeping the bedroom cool, dark, and quiet. By prioritizing sleep, individuals can boost their brain function, improve their overall health, and support their ability to learn and grow.

Engage in lifelong learning:
Keeping the mind active and engaged in learning new information and skills can help to keep the brain sharp and improve cognitive abilities.

Engaging in lifelong learning is a key way to keep the brain active and stimulated, and to boost cognitive abilities. Lifelong learning can take many forms, including taking classes, reading books, learning a new language, or picking up a new hobby. The act of learning new information and skills can help to challenge the brain and keep it active, which can slow down age-related declines in cognitive function.

Learning new information also creates new neural connections in the brain, which can help to improve memory, increase attention span, and boost overall cognitive abilities. In addition, engaging in lifelong learning can help to reduce stress, increase self-esteem, and provide a sense of purpose and fulfillment.

Lifelong learning can be accessible to anyone, at any age, and can be tailored to individual interests and needs. Whether through formal education or self-directed learning, the benefits of lifelong learning are numerous and can help to empower the human mind in meaningful ways. By keeping the mind active and engaged in learning, individuals can keep their brains sharp, boost their cognitive abilities, and continue to grow and evolve throughout their lives.

Brain plasticity refers to the ability of the brain to change and adapt in response to new experiences or information. This means that the brain can develop new connections and pathways in response to stimuli, which can help to improve brain function and cognitive abilities. Engaging in mentally stimulating activities and practicing mindfulness and meditation can help to build new connections in the brain and increase brain plasticity.

Examples of mentally challenging activities that can improve brain plasticity include Learning a new skill or language, Engaging in mentally challenging tasks such as puzzles, games, or memory exercises, Taking up a new hobby that requires cognitive effort and focus, Practicing mindfulness and meditation to improve focus and attention

Practice mindfulness and meditation:
Mindfulness and meditation practices have been shown to reduce stress, increase focus and attention, and boost emotional well-being. Practicing mindfulness and meditation is another key way to boost the human mind. These practices have been shown to have several benefits for mental health and well-being, including reducing stress, increasing focus and attention, and boosting emotional well-being.

Mindfulness involves paying attention to the present moment and being aware of your thoughts, feelings, and sensations. It can help to cultivate a non-judgmental attitude towards your experiences and can help to reduce feelings of stress, anxiety, and depression.

Meditation is a practice that involves focusing the mind and calming the body. It can help to increase attention and focus, reduce stress, and improve emotional well-being. There are many different types of meditation, including mindfulness meditation, guided meditation, and body scan meditation, among others.

Both mindfulness and meditation can be practiced anywhere and at any time, and do not require any special equipment or training. They can be incorporated into a daily routine and can provide a simple and accessible way to boost the human mind.

This principle of meditation and mindfulness revealed that through the intentional focus and concentration of meditation, we can quiet the mind, reduce stress and anxiety, and improve mental and physical health.

Meditation can involve a wide range of practices and techniques, including mindfulness meditation, mantra meditation, and body scan meditation, among others. The common denominator of these practices is the intentional focus and concentration on the present moment and not mindlessly opening your mind to something you do know. This could attract an unclean spirit into your life.

Research has shown that meditation can have several benefits, including reducing symptoms of anxiety and depression, improving sleep, boosting the immune system, and reducing chronic pain.[25] Meditation has also been shown to improve focus and attention, enhance creativity and problem-solving skills, and promote feelings of happiness and well-being.

---

[25] https://pubmed.ncbi.nlm.nih.gov/24395196/

The power of meditation can be used as a tool for enhancing mental and physical health and well-being. By incorporating meditation into our daily routine, we can reap the many benefits of this ancient practice, from reducing stress and anxiety to improving focus, creativity, and overall well-being.

The principle of meditation also highlights the importance of consistency and regular practice in achieving its full potential benefits. Research has shown that regular and consistent meditation practice, even for just a few minutes a day, can lead to long-term changes in brain structure and function.[26]

The practice of mindfulness and meditation can help to reduce stress, increase focus and attention, and boost emotional well-being. These practices can be easily incorporated into daily life and can provide a simple and effective way to boost the human mind and promote mental health and well-being.[27]

Meditation can also be a personal and introspective experience, helping individuals gain a deeper understanding of themselves, their emotions, and their thought patterns. It can promote self-awareness and increase emotional regulation, leading to better decision-making, improved relationships, and a more fulfilling life.

Moreover, meditation can be a holistic and inclusive practice, open to individuals of all cultures, backgrounds, and beliefs. It can be a tool for personal growth, self-discovery, and spiritual growth,

---

[26] https://pubmed.ncbi.nlm.nih.gov/26231761/
[27] https://pubmed.ncbi.nlm.nih.gov/27537781/

fostering a sense of connection and peace within the individual and the world around them.

In conclusion, the power of meditation highlights the potential of meditation as a tool for personal and spiritual growth enhanced mental and physical health, and overall well-being. By consistently and regularly incorporating meditation into our lives, we can tap into its full potential and reap its many benefits.

Stay socially connected:
Maintaining strong social connections has been linked to improved mental health, increased happiness, and improved cognitive function. Building strong relationships with others can provide support and stimulation, which can boost the mind and help individuals live a more fulfilling life.

Having strong social connections with friends, family, and others can provide a support network and a source of stimulation. Positive interactions with others can increase feelings of happiness and improve overall mental health. Studies have also shown that maintaining a strong social network can be beneficial for cognitive function, helping to keep the mind sharp.[28]

Participating in social activities, having meaningful conversations, and having positive relationships can all contribute to the boosting of your cognitive functions.[29]

---

[28] https://systematicreviewsjournal.biomedcentral.com/articles/10.1186/s13643-017-0632-2
[29] https://bmcgeriatr.biomedcentral.com/articles/10.1186/s12877-021-02531-0

Stay physically active:
Regular physical activity has been linked to improved cognitive function, increased energy, and reduced risk of depression and anxiety. Physical activity also provides a natural boost to brain function by increasing blood flow and oxygen to the brain.

Staying physically active is important for maintaining good mental health and overall well-being. Regular physical activity has been shown to improve cognitive function, including memory, attention, and problem-solving skills. This is because physical activity increases blood flow and oxygen to the brain, which can help to nourish and protect brain cells. Additionally, exercise releases endorphins, which are natural mood boosters that can improve overall mood and reduce stress and anxiety.

Physical activity can also provide a natural boost to energy levels, which can help to increase motivation and focus. Regular physical activity has been linked to reduced risk of depression and anxiety, as well as improved sleep quality, which can have a positive impact on mental health.

Overall, staying physically active can be a powerful tool for empowering and improving the human mind. Whether it's through structured exercise like running or playing sports, or simply by incorporating physical activity into daily life through activities like walking or gardening, making physical activity a regular part of life can help to boost mental well-being and improve cognitive function.

Nourish the body with healthy food:
Eating a balanced diet that is rich in fruits, vegetables, and whole grains can provide the brain with the nutrients it needs to function

at its best. A balanced diet that is rich in fruits, vegetables, and whole grains can provide the brain with the essential nutrients it needs to function optimally.

A diet that is high in processed foods and sugar, on the other hand, can negatively impact the brain, leading to decreased cognitive function, increased inflammation, and a greater risk of developing chronic health conditions. Some of the specific nutrients that are important for brain health include omega-3 fatty acids, vitamin B12, and antioxidants. By eating a well-balanced diet, individuals can provide their brain with the nutrients it needs to stay healthy and functioning at its best, which can help to boost the human mind.

Manage stress:
Chronic stress can have negative effects on the brain, including decreased memory and attention, and increased anxiety and depression. Effective stress management techniques, such as deep breathing, meditation, or exercise, can help to reduce stress and improve mental health.

Stress management is the process of identifying and reducing the sources of stress in one's life. It involves using various techniques to regulate the physiological and psychological responses to stress and to maintain a healthy balance between the demands of life and one's resources. Stress management can include a combination of lifestyle changes, such as exercise and relaxation techniques, as well as therapy, medication, or other forms of treatment.

When the brain experiences stress, it triggers the release of stress hormones, such as cortisol and adrenaline. In the short term, these hormones can improve focus and alertness. However, chronic stress can lead to a persistent elevation in cortisol levels, which can have negative effects on the brain, including decreased memory and attention, and increased anxiety and depression.

Effective stress management techniques can help to regulate the physiological stress response and reduce the negative effects of cortisol on the brain. By practicing relaxation techniques, such as deep breathing, and meditation, individuals can reduce their physiological stress response, and lower cortisol levels. In addition, engaging in regular exercise, eating a healthy diet, getting enough sleep, and engaging in mentally stimulating activities can help to build resilience to stress and improve overall mental health.

Additionally, practicing stress management techniques such as deep breathing, visualization, or physical activity can help reduce the negative impact of stress on the mind. Challenging the brain with new and engaging activities like puzzles, games, or new hobbies can also stimulate the brain and keep it functioning at its best. Taking time to engage in hobbies and interests that bring joy and fulfillment can help to boost mood and improve overall mental health. Finally, setting and working towards meaningful goals can provide a sense of purpose and direction, which can be empowering and positively influence the mind.

Focus on positivity:
Cultivating a positive outlook and focusing on the good in life has been linked to improved mental well-being, increased happiness, and improved cognitive function.

Focus on positivity refers to the intentional practice of paying attention to the positive aspects of life, and actively seeking out opportunities to see the good in people, situations, and experiences.

Fostering a positive outlook has been shown to have a significant impact on mental health and cognitive function. Research has found that people with a positive outlook tend to experience lower levels of stress, anxiety, and depression, and higher levels of happiness and life satisfaction. Additionally, positive thinking has been linked to improved cognitive function, including increased focus and attention, and improved memory.

One of the ways that positivity can influence the brain is by reducing the impact of stress. Chronic stress has been linked to a variety of negative effects on the brain, including decreased memory and attention, and increased anxiety and depression.[30] [31] By focusing on the positive aspects of life, individuals can reduce the amount of stress they experience, and thereby mitigate the negative impact that stress can have on the brain.

Furthermore, focusing on positivity can help to build new connections in the brain, and increase brain plasticity. Brain plasticity refers to the ability of the brain to change and adapt in response to new experiences, information, and stimuli. Engaging in positive thinking and experiences can help to create new neural connections in the brain, leading to improved cognitive function and greater overall brain health.

---

[30] https://www.tuw.edu/health/how-stress-affects-the-brain/
[31] https://theconversation.com/how-chronic-stress-changes-the-brain-and-what-you-can-do-to-reverse-the-damage-133194

THE METAMORPHOSIS OF THE MIND

Chapter 18

The Spiritual Dimensions of Mental Wellness

Some spirituality activities can help you with anxiety, depression, suicide, and hopelessness. Spiritual practices refer to activities or rituals that are undertaken to cultivate a deeper connection with the spiritual aspects of life, self, or a higher power. These practices are often rooted in religious traditions, but they can also be pursued independently or as part of a broader spiritual philosophy.

According to various studies, attending church may offer benefits in terms of reducing stress and enhancing happiness. However, there is a difference between being religious and being spiritual. Neal Krause and colleagues' research indicates that individuals identifying as "religious" reported a higher prevalence of health-related problems compared to those who identified as "spiritual," "religious and spiritual," or "neither religious nor spiritual." This observation prompts Krause to put forth an intriguing perspective on the relationship between religion and spirituality.

Krause suggests that spirituality is not contradictory to religion but, instead, serves as the emotional essence or soul of religious practices. In other words, he posits that the emotional and experiential elements associated with spirituality are fundamental to the overall well-being of individuals within a religious context.

The statement implies that engaging in religious rituals without a genuine and emotionally connected spiritual experience may render those rituals sterile and impersonal. In Krause's view, spirituality is not an opposing force to religious practices; rather, it brings depth and vitality to these practices by infusing them with emotional significance. The essence of this perspective is that a more profound spiritual engagement enhances the positive impact of religious activities on an individual's health and overall sense of well-being.

Therefore, according to Krause, it is not merely the identification as "religious" that influences health outcomes, but the presence of meaningful and experiential spirituality within religious practices that plays a crucial role in promoting positive health and well-being. This viewpoint encourages a deeper exploration of the emotional and spiritual dimensions within religious frameworks to better understand their potential impact on individuals' physical and mental health.[32][33]

---

[32] Neal Krause, Kenneth I. Pargament, Peter C. Hill, & Gail Ironson. (2019a). *Exploring religious and/or spiritual identities: Part 1 - Assessing relationships with health. Mental Health, Religion, & Culture,* 22 (9), 877-891.

[33] Neal Krause, Kenneth I. Pargament, Peter C. Hill, & Gail Ironson. (2019b). *Exploring religious and/or spiritual identities: Part 2 - A descriptive analysis of those who are at risk for health problems. Mental Health, Religion, & Culture,* 22 (9), 892-909.

Here are some potent spiritual practices:
Prayer: Many people find comfort, inspiration, and hope in prayer. Prayer is a way of communicating and communing with God. It can be done in silence, aloud, or in writing. Prayer can help you express your gratitude, praise, confession, requests, or intercession to God. Prayer can also help you listen to God's voice and guidance in your life.

Prayers can take various forms, including personal and informal conversations with a higher power, recitation of Scriptural texts, or participation in organized religious services. People engage in prayer for spiritual connection, guidance, and comfort, or as a way of expressing faith and devotion. It is a common practice in many religious and spiritual traditions and is considered a means of seeking solace, strength, and a deeper understanding of one's beliefs.

Worship: Worship is a way of honoring and praising God for who he is and what he has done. It can be done individually or communally, through singing, music, dancing, art, or other forms of expression. Worship can help you celebrate God's goodness, grace, and love. It can also help you connect with God's presence and power.

Fasting: Fasting is the voluntary abstention from food, drink, or certain activities for a specific period. It is often undertaken for religious, spiritual, or health reasons. Fasting can take various forms, such as intermittent fasting, water fasting, or abstaining from specific types of food. Many cultures and religions incorporate fasting into their practices as a means of self-discipline, purification, or spiritual reflection. In addition to its spiritual significance, some individuals adopt fasting for potential health benefits, such as improved metabolism and detoxification.

Reading/Studying: Reading or studying scriptures involves engaging with sacred texts. This practice aims to gain knowledge, insight, and spiritual guidance from these texts. People often turn to scriptures to deepen their understanding of religious teachings, moral principles, and the nature of existence. This practice can involve individual study, group discussions, or attending religious services where scriptures are read and interpreted. It plays a central role in many religious traditions as a means of fostering spiritual growth, moral development, and a connection with divine wisdom. Bible reading and meditation are ways of studying and reflecting on God's word. They can help you understand God's character, will, and plan for you. They can also help you apply God's word to your daily life and challenges.

Forgiveness: Forgiveness is the act of pardoning or letting go of resentment and bitterness towards someone who has wronged or hurt you. It involves releasing negative emotions, seeking understanding, and choosing not to hold onto anger or a desire for revenge. Forgiveness can contribute to personal healing, promote reconciliation, and allow for emotional and spiritual growth. It is a powerful and transformative process that often benefits both the forgiver and the forgiven.

Benefits of forgiveness:
Forgiveness involves letting go of resentment, anger, and negative emotions towards the person who caused harm. This release of emotional burden can lead to a sense of relief, reducing stress and promoting emotional well-being.

Forgiveness allows individuals to address and heal emotional wounds caused by past hurts. By acknowledging the pain and choosing to forgive, individuals can take steps toward inner healing and find closure to emotional injuries.

Forgiveness is a crucial element in the process of reconciliation. When individuals forgive and are forgiven, it creates an opportunity to rebuild trust and restore relationships. Open communication, empathy, and understanding often follow forgiveness, fostering a sense of connection.

Forgiveness disrupts the cycle of retaliation and revenge. Instead of perpetuating negative actions, forgiving individuals choose a path of understanding and compassion, contributing to a more positive and harmonious social environment.

Forgiveness often involves understanding the perspective of the wrongdoer. This empathetic approach not only contributes to forgiveness but also nurtures a deeper understanding of others, promoting compassion and empathy in relationships.

Choosing forgiveness requires a level of emotional maturity and self-reflection. It allows individuals to learn from their experiences, cultivate resilience, and develop a greater sense of self-awareness. This process contributes to personal growth and increases emotional intelligence.

Forgiveness is a central theme in many spiritual and religious traditions. By forgiving, individuals align with principles of compassion, mercy, and love, fostering spiritual growth and a sense of inner peace.

Holding onto grudges can lead to bitterness and a negative outlook on life. Forgiveness helps in releasing these negative emotions, creating space for positive emotions, joy, and a more optimistic worldview.

Forgiveness is a transformative process that goes beyond merely pardoning someone. It involves emotional release, healing, restoration of relationships, and personal growth. By choosing forgiveness, individuals contribute to their well-being, promote harmony in relationships, and experience profound emotional and spiritual growth.

Simplicity and Acts of Service: Simplicity and acts of service are intertwined concepts that emphasize a humble and selfless approach to life. Simplicity involves a mindset of minimizing material attachments and living with a focus on essential values. It is about embracing a straightforward and uncluttered lifestyle, prioritizing meaningful connections over material possessions. Acts of service refer to selfless actions performed to benefit others. This can include helping those in need, contributing to the community, or supporting individuals facing challenges. Acts of service are motivated by compassion, empathy, and a desire to make a positive impact on the lives of others.

The connection between simplicity and acts of service lies in their shared emphasis on a selfless and purposeful life. Simplicity encourages individuals to be content with less and to channel their focus away from material accumulation. Acts of service complement this by directing attention towards the well-being and needs of others.

By embracing simplicity, individuals often find themselves with more time, resources, and mental space to engage in acts of service. Conversely, acts of service can reinforce the values of simplicity by highlighting the fulfillment that comes from contributing to the welfare of others rather than pursuing excessive material wealth. Together, simplicity and acts of service create a harmonious approach to life—one that values relationships, empathy, and a commitment to making a positive difference in the world.

Community Worship: Community worship involves gathering as a group to participate in spiritual activities or ceremonies. This collective practice fosters a sense of shared faith and connection among individuals within a community. Community worship plays a crucial role in reinforcing the shared identity of a religious or spiritual community. It provides a space for collective expression, mutual support, and the affirmation of common beliefs. It also often serves as a focal point for individuals to come together, fostering a sense of belonging and shared purpose.

During community worship, communities often come together for organized religious services, which may include prayers, hymns, sermons, and other ceremonies based on the specific religious tradition. Special occasions, festivals, or religious holidays are often marked with community worship, where members join in communal expressions of faith, gratitude, and celebration.

Community worship provides an opportunity for the dissemination of religious teachings, moral values, and spiritual insights. It often includes the reading or recitation of sacred texts and the sharing of wisdom. Beyond the religious aspects, community worship allows individuals to connect with others who share similar beliefs, fostering a supportive and communal environment. In many religious communities, individuals gather in circles for group prayers. This collective act of prayer is believed to amplify spiritual energy and create a sense of unity.

Marino Bruce, a Vanderbilt University professor and associate director of the school's Center For Research On Men's Health, discovered in a study published in the journal PLOS (Public Library Of Science) that people who attend worship services may reduce their mortality risk by 55 percent, particularly those aged 40 to 65.[34] Neal Krause, Ph.D., is the University of Michigan School of Public Health's Marshall H. Becker Collegiate Professor Emeritus. Neal has researched and written extensively on the relationship between religion and health in elderly individuals. For his studies, he has won numerous awards.

According to some web sources, going to church may have some benefits for reducing stress and improving happiness. However, these benefits may depend on various factors, such as the frequency, quality, and motivation of church attendance, as well as the individual's personal beliefs, preferences, and experiences. Going to church may not be the only or the best way to achieve happiness and well-being for everyone.

---

[34] Church attendance, allostatic load and mortality in middle-aged adults | PLOS ONE

Ultimately, the decision to go to church is a personal one that should be based on your faith, convictions, and needs.[35] [36] [37]

Meditation: Meditation is a practice that involves focused attention, mindfulness, or contemplation to achieve a state of inner calm, mental clarity, and heightened awareness. It often includes techniques such as deep breathing, guided visualization, or repeating mantras. Meditation is used for various purposes, including reducing stress, improving concentration, promoting emotional well-being, and exploring a deeper connection with oneself or spiritual dimensions. Regular meditation is associated with numerous physical and mental health benefits, making it a widely adopted practice for enhancing overall well-being.

"Meditating on the word of God" is the practice of deeply reflecting, contemplating, and pondering the holy scriptures. It involves deliberately focusing one's thoughts, attention, and contemplative energy on the teachings, verses, or passages of the holy scriptures, seeking to gain spiritual insight, understanding, and connection.

In Christianity, for example, the term often specifically refers to reflecting on the teachings and messages found in the Bible. This process of meditation typically involves more than just reading the words; it encompasses a thoughtful and intentional consideration of the meaning, relevance, and personal application of the scriptures. It goes beyond intellectual understanding to engage the heart, soul, and spirit in a profound exploration of one's faith.

---

[35] How Religion and Spirituality Affect Stress and Health | Psychology Today
[36] Going To Church Reduces Stress And Mortality - AnxietyCentre.com
[37] How Religion Can Improve on Your Mental Health (aarp.org)

Meditating on the word of God may involve various approaches, such as Repetition, Contemplation, Prayerful Reflection, and Application in one's daily life. It is a means of spiritual growth, deepening one's relationship with the divine, and gaining wisdom from the holy scriptures. It is a contemplative exercise that encourages believers to go beyond surface-level understanding and engage in a profound exploration of the spiritual truths contained in their religious scriptures.

Controversial Spiritual Practices:
Yoga: Yoga is a physical, mental, and spiritual practice that combines postures, breath control, and meditation to promote overall well-being and spiritual growth. However, some people believe that *yoga is a form of syncretism or compromise* since it mixes elements of different religions and spiritualities. According to some Medical Humanities, yoga is a form of syncretism or compromise, but a unique and independent practice that can be done for good or evil, depending on the user's intention and attitude. They also point out that yoga is not a monolithic phenomenon, but a diverse and evolving practice that can be adapted to different contexts and cultures.[38]

Some people believe that *yoga is a form of idolatry or worship of other gods* since it involves postures and gestures that are associated with Hindu deities and concepts. According to some web sources,

---

[38] Supple bodies, healthy minds: yoga, psychedelics and American mental health | Medical Humanities (bmj.com)

yoga poses are seen as acts of idolatry that produce a force known as the serpent power, which is of occult origin.[39]

Some people believe that *yoga is a form of occultism or witchcraft* since it involves meditation, chanting, and energy manipulation that may open doors to demonic influences. According to The Guardian, yoga is a form of occultism or witchcraft, since it is based on ancient pagan teachings and practices. [Chris Flanders, Fri 26 Jun 2020 10.00 BST Last modified on Fri 26 Jun 2020 14.05 BST.[40]

Other controversial practices include:
Yoga: Tiara Isabella's article on the Vox website, published on February 3, 2018, highlighted a controversy surrounding yoga. Entitled "A Catholic blogger says Christians shouldn't do yoga. Does he have a point?" it referenced a Twitter post by Matt Walsh of The Daily Wire, drawing parallels between yoga and occult practices such as Ouija boards.[41] This viewpoint has been echoed across platforms like Reddit[42] and other social media, suggesting that yoga poses serve as a conduit for demonic influence and interaction.

Ultimately, the decision to practice yoga or not is a personal one that should be based on one's conscience, values, and understanding. Therefore, it is important to do one's research, ask

---

[39] https://www.thetruelight.net/wp/10-yoga-poses-that-offer-worship-to-hindu-deities/;https://capro.info/yoga-mindless-idolatry/; https://www.womenofgrace.com:8443/blog/?p=72450.

[40] Experience: my yoga class turned out to be a cult | Life and style | The Guardian

[41] A Catholic blogger says Christians shouldn't do yoga. Does he have a point? - Vox

[42] Why do people say yoga is satanic? : r/yoga (reddit.com)

questions, consult with trusted and knowledgeable people, and pray for guidance before making a choice.

Chanting and Mantras: Repetitive vocalizations of sacred sounds or phrases believed to have spiritual significance, promoting focus and spiritual connection.

Contemplative Walks: Walking with a focused and meditative mindset, often in nature, to connect with the environment and one's inner self.

Rituals and Ceremonies: Formalized practices with symbolic significance, often associated with religious traditions. In some occult or esoteric traditions, rituals may involve animal sacrifice as a symbolic or ritualistic act believed to channel spiritual energies, gain favor from deities, or achieve specific magical purposes. According to Thane Grauel, an Occult expert finds the black magic in animal killings in his USA Today's, The (Westchester County, N.Y.) Journal News, suggests that there are some practices and traditions that involve killing animals for occult or religious purposes.[43]

---

[43] Occult expert finds the black magic in animal killings (usatoday.com)

Epilogue

Dear Esteemed Readers,

As you have come to the final pages of "The Metamorphosis of the Mind," I invite you to reflect upon the profound exploration that has woven the fabric of your understanding. You have traversed the diverse landscapes of psychology, philosophy, and theology, unraveling the intricate nature of the mind's triad nature and strategies for winning the internal wars.

I wish to express my heartfelt appreciation for the resilience within you, a force that emerged from the depths of your shared exploration. It is this resilience that has enabled you to navigate the complex realms of the mind, confront challenges, and embrace the transformative power of positive thinking.

As you close this chapter and move forward, may this epilogue stand as a beacon of encouragement. Your journey towards perpetual metamorphosis is a testament to the strength within. Embrace the ongoing transformation of your mind, nurture the seeds of positivity, and continue to embark on the path of growth. With deepest gratitude and warm regards,

Elisha O. Ogbonna
https://www.elishaogbonna.com/

Other Books

Mastering the Power of Your Emotions: *How to control what happens in you irrespective of what happens in you* - Copyright © June 7, 2021, by Elisha O. Ogbonna

Every day of our lives, we are faced with situations that could bring to us joy or sadness, love or hatred, fear or confidence. Every event and obstacle of the world around us aims at taking hold of our emotions to influence our feelings and actions.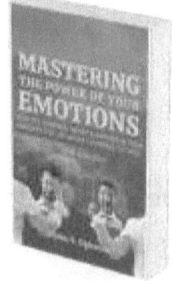

In mastering the power of your emotions, you will be presented with an instructive map of the emotional landscapes that many of us are forced to navigate. You will learn the five laws of emotions and discover:

- How temperament and character influence our emotional responses;
- How to respond rather than react to a situation;
- How to handle rejection, abandonment, depression, and grief;
- How to navigate through suicidal thoughts and self-harm behaviours;
- How to handle anonymous threats and various emotional crises;
- How to gain confidence and have a good self-image;
- How to release and replace negative emotions with positive ones

... and a lot more.

A useful, upbeat, and well-organized guide to managing emotions and building resilience and strength... (Kirkus Review March 30, 2018)

Mastering Frustration – Elisha O. Ogbonna

Do you feel like your goals are always out of reach? Does your job make you tear your hair out? Are you fed up with dead-end relationships? Discover a practical method to turn stress into satisfaction.

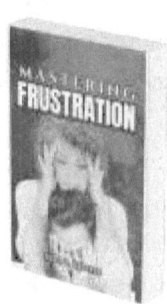

Mastering Frustration is a hands-on approach to conquering everyday fears, annoyances, or challenges that can end up ruining your world. Divided into three specific areas of Personal, Occupational, and Home, Ogbonna provides guidelines for resolving a wide span of issues. By handling your obstacles and stresses, you'll soon be building a bridge back to the happy life you deserve.

In *Mastering Frustration*, you'll discover:
- Tools and techniques to change unfavorable situations into fulfilling experiences
- How to triumph over the damaging effects of despair, sadness, and depression and find your true resilience
- Ways to create permission for yourself to transform unhealthy scenarios into positive outcomes
- Specific turning points to give you leverage over the changes you desire
- Helpful descriptions of problems, identifying persistent sources of aggravation, actionable steps, and much, much more!

Mastering Frustration is a detailed guide to help you regain sanity. If you like expert assistance, pragmatic strategies, and easy-to-follow advice, then you'll love Elisha O. Ogbonna's game-changing resource.

Get *Mastering Frustration* to turn your tension into hope today!

Empowered Thinking: *The Pathway to Self-Discovery and Fulfillment* – Elisha O. Ogbonna

Embark on a transformative journey of self-discovery and empowerment with "Empowered Thinking." In this enlightening guide, Elisha O. Ogbonna delves into the profound exploration of intricate thoughts, thought patterns, and the relationship between the human mind and the transformative force of positive thinking.

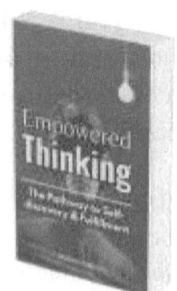

Unlike generic self-help books, "Empowered Thinking" offers factual and practical insights for individuals grappling with self-identity, self-discovery, and mental challenges such as indecision, overthinking, confusion, doubt, unbelief, and impacts from discouraging experiences.

As readers progress, they explore "The Act of Thinking," delving into thought patterns, sources of thoughts, and practical tools for cultivating positivity. The guide introduces the 5P's of shattering mental barricades, distinguishing between changeable and unchangeable aspects of life, and deconstructing cognitive obstacles for a liberated mindset.

Ogbonna presents "Thinking the Right Thoughts" as a strategic blueprint for transcending self-limiting paradigms, urging readers to contemplate broader perspectives on thinking beyond self, fear, size, and societal influence.

This book is not just a guide; it's a transformative roadmap to self-discovery and fulfillment. Elisha Ogbonna equips readers with the knowledge to navigate challenges and embrace positivity for lasting transformation. "Empowered Thinking" is a must-read for anyone seeking to unleash their inner potential and live a life of purpose and meaning.

Mastering Success: *How to get to the top and remain there* – Elisha O. Ogbonna

Looking to turn those good intentions into amazing results? Learn how to discover your inner wisdom to create the life of your dreams.

Do you continually hit frustrating hurdles? Does your existence seem stuck at a crossroads? Confused about which direction to take to drive better outcomes? Author, teacher, business leader, and speaker Elisha O. Ogbonna has on-the-ground experience in turning stagnant organizations and their people around to achieve their objectives. Now he's here to share his system for creating breakthroughs so you can reach the pinnacle of your game... without falling back down.

Mastering Success: How to Get to the Top and Remain There is a powerful guide to discovering your perfect fulfillment. Set out in five specific parts that take you through self-discovery and goal-setting strategies, Ogbonna supplies growth and sustainability techniques applicable to every aspect of your life. By following these practical methods, you'll unlock your dream purpose and nail your accomplishments with a winner's ease.

In *Mastering Success*, you'll discover:
- The key principles of self-development to unleash your hidden powers
- How to set goals to make great results inevitable
- Ways to build community and partnerships to leverage your productivity
- Methods to develop resilience and maintain your focus on peace and happiness
- Tactics for those just starting their journey, ego traps to avoid, business applications, and much, much more!

Mastering Success is a detailed and effective manual to help anyone forge their future. If you like dynamic thinking, transformational tools, and down-to-earth advice, then you'll love Elisha O. Ogbonna's outstanding resource.

Get *Mastering Success* to climb your mountain today!

www.ingramcontent.com/pod-product-compliance
Lightning Source LLC
Chambersburg PA
CBHW022057160426
43198CB00008B/263